# How to be Healthy and Live Longer

# How to be Healthy and Live Longer

*A guidebook to vitality and health through
physical and mental development
and a natural foods diet.*

By

John H. Tobe

## Greywood Publishing Limited

101 Duncan Mill Road • Don Mills, Ontario

# CONTENTS

# INTRODUCTION

Does there exist a greater goal in life for any man than to live long in good health, physically and mentally?

The very simple basic fact that we have been allowed a niche on this earth should indicate clearly and unmistakably that it is our duty and purpose to live in it in good health as long as humanly possible.

It is only by making full use of our faculties that we can fulfil our mission on earth. I contend the greatest achievements on earth were accomplished by men in good health. The evil that has been wrought upon mankind was concocted by men who were sick mentally or physically.

I contend that the goal of good health and long life is more important than spiritual, familial, sensual and financial goals because these have no meaning without health and long years of life.

Then and only then can you go on to achieve greatness in the spiritual or other lines of human relations and endeavours. Therefore, I maintain that the aim towards long life in good health is the highest and noblest goal to which a human being can aspire.

Of what value is success, or renown, or greatness, without good health? None! Therefore, I admonish you, I urge you, I beseech you ... first and foremost strive to achieve good health.

# CHAPTER 1

## Road to Long Life

*To me, there is no more important endeavour in life than to plan, work and aspire to live long — and to live free from the tyranny of disease. The value of health is far above that of financial achievement, social success or political freedom. After all, there is no bondage so fearful, no poverty so cruel, no failure so unhappy as that encompassed by the word sickness.*

. . . . DR. VICTOR H. LANDLAHR.

### YOU CAN LIVE TO BE ONE HUNDRED

I maintain that it is the inherent right of every human being to live to be at least one hundred years of age.

I'm not going into a long discussion as to how long a human being can live, for in truth nobody really knows. But the fact is that hundreds of thousands of people throughout the world live to be one hundred years of age and more and there are records that prove that even ages of 150 and 200 are not impossible.

I solemnly stand before you and say that because hundreds of thousands of people have lived and are living to be more than one hundred years of age, you can do it too. Do you have the will, the determination, the strength of character to achieve this inherent right of every human being? Of course, I am fully aware of the fact that you did not gain sufficient knowledge early enough in life but nevertheless, you can as of this day begin to improve your health and add to your years by following the principles as outlined here in this volume.

Students of longevity calculate that animals live to be approximately seven times their maturity age.

Whether we like it or not, man is, according to biological concepts, an animal. The point is how do we judge the age of maturity of 'homo sapiens'? Do we judge it by sexual maturity? Or by the ability to perform physical labor? Or by mental maturity? Depending upon the accepted type of maturity, these ages would vary from about 14 to 21 years.

11

The latter is the legal age of maturity for the male of the species. Now multiply the above ages by seven and we get 98 to 147 years. Therefore, no matter how you figure it, a man ought to live at least 100 years in sound health.

May I offer a simple analogy as proof of my contention that you can add years of life even though you have a record of over-indulgence? You are all familiar with the proverbial case of the straw that broke the camel's back. If you keep loading the camel straw upon straw, there will come a time when one straw will be the actual cause of breaking the back of the camel . . . and if continued, the camel will be destroyed.

On the other hand, if you only come close to this destructive point and you begin to remove straws singly, soon the camel will, with each straw that is removed, become stronger and will stand erect again.

Therefore, I maintain that if you start as of now to correct the errors in your pattern of living you can quickly move towards an improvement in your physical condition and this, of itself, must give you added moments, hours, days and years of life.

Therefore, I reiterate . . . you can live to be one hundred and more than one hundred. If you are young and have not seriously damaged your body, if you have had no organs removed and have your teeth or most of them, then your chances of reaching the century mark and beyond are excellent.

I do not have to point out to you that over-indulgence in smoking, drinking and the eating of improper foods will shorten your life and if you have indulged in these, then you have done some greater or lesser harm to your body. But the harm of these evils can be alleviated, if not to a great extent overcome. Furthermore, I do not suggest that making the transition is easy. But first you must break these harmful habits to which you are addicted.

In making the changeover you are actually eating better foods, more wholesome foods and more palatable foods, but because of habit and our perverted tastes, we often do not recognize this until months or sometimes even a year

12

or two after we have made the transition. The changeover is basically simple if we have the strength of character to see and to recognize it in its cold stark nakedness. But our unhealthy eating habits in most cases blind us to the truth and make us believe that it is a great effort and a big sacrifice to give up the evils and take on the delights and pleasures of life to be found in eating proper natural foods.

## ANYTHING YOU CAN DO
## I CAN DO ... BETTER

I don't know how you feel about man's achievements but I've always felt that what one man could do, another could do better. I will admit that Shakespeares or his kind don't crop up every day but there will be someone as great or greater in the near or distant future who will do better. I am not writing this to decry Shakespeare's genius, but what I am trying to convey to you is the fact that what one man has accomplished another man can equal or improve upon. I admit that it may take effort, time and study but I firmly reiterate ... that what one man has achieved you, too, can accomplish.

At the conclusion of this article I am going to give you a list of people who have lived beyond the one hundred mark.

While writing this book one of the titles that seemed suitable was, "You Can Live to be Over One Hundred Years Old." Then it struck me that living to be one hundred or more was not the big or the main achievement, but living to be one hundred in good health and sound mentality ... well, that is something worthwhile.

I am sure that we all have known many people who have lived to be 70, 80 and 90 and beyond but they were sick, ailing, doddery, senile or half alive. Unless one can live to a ripe old age in good health and mentality, I do not consider it a bargain.

In a volume written by John Smith called, "The Natural Food of Man", Sir William Temple is quoted as stating that back in the 16th Century when the Europeans first discovered Central and South America they found the natives of those tropical regions had a life span of over 200 years.

Now in giving you the list that follows I want you to know that I just compiled it from various, easily available sources without attempting by any means to give you a broad list of those who lived to be over one hundred, because there were and are thousands of people who have exceeded the age of one hundred years. What others have done, you can equal or better.

Here is the list of notables and plain people who found life good and learned how to extend their years to heights unknown today:

Sadhu Swami, Karimganji, India, was reported to be 330 years old in 1923.

Li Chung-yun, China, died in 1933 at the age of 256.

Sayed Ali, Kelusah, Persia, was 195 years old in 1962.

Petraz Czarten died in Kopros, Hungary in 1724 at the age of 185 years.

Mrs. Maria Garzon Ciuda de Castaneda, Colombia, 178 years in 1956.

Javier Pereira, Colombia, was between 155 and 166 years in 1965.

William Bisset, Port Elizabeth, South Africa, was 160 in 1956.

Joseph Surrington died in a village near Bergen in 1797 at the age of 160.

Shiralibaba Muslimov, a Russian living in a mountain village in Azerbaijan, was 160 years old in 1965.

Thomas Parr lived to 153 years of age . . . died in 1635.

Lyubov Puka, a Russian, claims to be 150 years old. He has two younger brothers, aged 120 and 118, and a sister 112.

Mahmud Fivozov, Azerbaijan Republic, bordering Iran, was 147 in 1955.

Drakenberg, a Dane, lived 146 years.

Galen, the great physician, lived 140 years.

H. Jenkins, from Yorkshire, was a witness in court for a happening 140 years before. His two sons, 100 and 102 years of age, accompanied him.

14

John Bayley, Northampton, died at 130 years.

Moses — 127 years.

Peter Albrecht lived to be 123 years old.

Sayed Ali's eldest son died at 120, two sons are 105 and 90 and a daughter is 110.

Gurgen Doublas of Sweden reached 120 years.

Jean Thuret's mother died at 118 and his uncle at 130.

Maria Willamow, St. Petersburg, died in 1807 at 115 years of age.

Walter W. William celebrated his 114th birthday in 1956.

R. Glan, Philadelphia, Pa., died in 1796 at the age of 114.

Joseph — 110 years.

Dado, citizen of Hunza, was 110 in 1965.

Maria Willamow's brother predeceased her in 1768 at the age of 108.

Baron Baravicino de Capellis, an Italian, died in 1770 in his 107th year.

Mrs. William Miller, Hollywood, Florida was 107 in 1956.

Mrs. Laura Stantson, La Grange, Georgia, died at 106 in 1956.

Peter V. Ortiz, Anaheim, California, was 106 years old in 1956.

Jean Thuret lived beyond the age of 104.

Midwife who attended Henrietta Maria, wife of Charles I, lived to be 103.

Mrs. de Vere of Canterbury, Britain, was 103 in 1961.

Amos Alonzo Stagg, American football coach, died in 1965 at age 102.

## YOU CAN GROW YOUNGER

Fifteen years ago if someone had told me or I had read somewhere an article saying, "You can grow younger," I would have snorted, "Bunk! Baloney! Who do they think they're trying to fool?"

Yet today I find myself writing a section of my book and giving it that title . . . and the incredible part of it, even to me, is the simple straightforward fact that you *can* grow younger. Therefore, I'm not going to mince matters — I'm going to get right down to facts and give you some case histories.

As of this hour these people are alive and healthier than they have ever been and are ready to bear witness that what I say is true. I have selected ten because I don't have room for any more. But these ten were chosen from a list of more than twenty-five that I have in my files and it is available for anyone's scrutiny.

So if you want proof that you can grow younger, read on ...

### William Langmuir

I have known this man for about ten years. During these ten years this man has grown younger. He looks and is healthier at 75 than he was at 65. Here is the gist of his story:

"At fifty-five I was a sick man, ailing in all parts of my body. I felt that the best I could hope for, if lucky, was a few more years of invalidism. Then my wife died. Shortly after that I began to live. Now don't get me wrong. I loved my wife very much — she was a wonderful woman — but she was killing me with kindness and her cooking.

"After her death I began to read and study health and nutrition. Then I began to eat according to the knowledge that I had gained. I ate what I wanted and when I wanted it. I have continued in this manner right up to the present time.

"I changed my entire method of eating, following chiefly the practices of natural hygiene and today my diet consists almost entirely of unfired foods. I attest to the fact that at 75 I am a much healthier man ... in fact, I am in practically perfect condition ... whereas at 55 I was ailing and dying."

This selfsame youngster of 75 came into our establishment some time ago carrying a 30-lb. pail of honey in each hand and walking briskly and erectly. His skin is as clear as a baby's, his eyes sparkle and his walk is as firm and solid as that of a guardsman. He is truly a better physical specimen at 75 than most men of 40 or 50. He told me

16

recently that he had visited an optometrist for a routine eye examination and was told that he no longer needed his glasses.

## Ted Arbuthnot

This chap came to see me first about three years ago. He said he'd like to meet me and talk to me. He informed me that he had had a bad heart attack and had been told that he'd have to take it easy for the rest of his days.

He went on to say, "I'd like to know more about food and its effect upon health. Will you suggest some reading material for me?"

I scanned the list of six hundred or so titles that we have and made a selection for him. We discussed food and diet for some time and then he took his leave.

He comes back every few months and selects further reading matter and we have a good chat. He is back at his work full time and is the picture of good health. He is a handsome man, anyway, and he states emphatically, "I never felt better in my life. I feel as though I'm getting younger every day."

He also told me that he has changed his entire mode of eating and living, is taking regular exercise, and right now he has the body of a topnotch athlete.

The other day he said to me, "I am thinking seriously of retiring to a farm or a piece of land where I really can work." He feels that he wants to devote himself to a life of greater physical activity.

I wholeheartedly applauded the idea.

## Richard Percival

When I first knew Percival he drank, smoked and ate without restriction or reservation. His general appearance and actions did not reflect good health. He appeared quarrelsome and discontented.

When he first came to the establishment he didn't ask my advice — he just browsed around the bookshelves from time to time, selecting and purchasing various titles. Later, we began to converse and get to know each other.

17

This has been going on now for six or seven years and he, more than anyone else, has paralleled my own serious and protracted attempt to acquire knowledge. He no longer drinks or smokes, his disposition has improved and so has his general outlook on life. He follows a diet pattern based on the knowledge he has gained and today in his middle sixties he is a much younger man than he was when I first knew him.

He doesn't know what an ache or pain means. He hasn't had a cold or missed a day's work in years ... at least since he started on this way of life. Seven years have gone by since he saw the first ray of light and he is younger today than he was seven years ago.

## Leonard Orville

Orville is a high school teacher. He is about as pleasant and even tempered a human being as you will find in a lifetime ... a genuine intellectual, a wonderful teacher, a fine father, a good husband and a splendid friend.

Three years ago he had a heart attack. After he had recovered sufficiently to get around again, I said to him one day, "How would you like it if you could once and for all banish the fear of ever having another attack?"

He replied, "That would be wonderful if it were possible!"

"Well," I said, "it surely is ... just as sure as the sun rises and sets! Are you interested?"

"Yes, most assuredly," he replied.

So I began to direct him along the road to knowledge on food, nutrition, health and diet. Today he is as well informed as any man I know. His diet consists almost entirely of unfired foods. He has lost about fifteen pounds and is as slender and agile as a lad of sixteen, has a good complexion, splendid tone, gleaming eyes. Last summer he played basketball and baseball.

In my estimation he is ten years younger than he was when he had his heart attack. He is in perfect physical condition.

18

*John H. Tobe*

I think that these case histories should include my own. Up until the time I was thirty-nine I considered myself to be in almost perfect health. Then one day I found that I was losing my sexual virility. That started me on my quest for youth. The only difference between Ponce de Leon and me is that I found it . . . for at sixty-five I am a better man than I was at thirty-nine.

Furthermore, I do at least three times as much work at sixty-five as I did at thirty-nine and I am increasing my output rather than decreasing it. I feel neither aches nor pains. I use glasses only where the light is poor. I work fifteen hours every day, including Sundays when I devote myself mainly to reading and studying.

I know I am younger at sixty-five than I was at thirty-nine.

*Grace Fraser*

This girl has been an employee of mine for sixteen years. During the first few years she worked for me she would take time off every now and then to visit her doctor. She was bothered with various female complaints and these signs of degeneration persisted until a couple of years ago when she swung over sharply to the hygienic way of living . . . existing chiefly on uncooked foods . . . vegetable salads, grains, fruits and nuts, with a strict minimum of cooked foods.

There is no doubt about it, at forty-four years of age she is a much younger woman than she was at twenty-eight. She has a step as spry as a girl of sixteen, her mind is as keen as a razor, her eyes are as sharp as those of a hawk, and she moves about and bristles like static electricity.

*Alice Landry*

This lady is now seventy-eight years of age. At seventy-seven she had a heart attack. Her family did not expect her to live very long . . . it looked like the end. She had a very bad eye condition as well as edema which caused her legs to swell out of all proportion. She liked her coffee and drank enormous quantities of it.

For the past six months she has switched over almost entirely to an unfired food diet and she looks years younger than she did a year ago. All of the conditions have shown marked improvement and some have completely disappeared. The change in this old lady would have to be seen to be believed . . . and all in the space of less than a year! I predict that next year she'll be younger and spryer than ever.

## Charlie Griffiths

He came in to see me about three years ago. He looked around, bought a few of our natural foods, and then inquired about a juicer. It didn't take him long to negotiate a deal and he walked out with a few natural food items, a juicer and a few books that he had selected.

From then on he came back every second week for grains and dried fruits and he always browsed around the bookshelves and picked up a few books.

The other day I discussed with him his case history. I wanted to know more about him. First, he told me that he is sixty years old. About three years ago he had had a big lump in his groin . . . bigger than a golf ball.

He went to his physician who recommended surgery. This he refused. He had great trouble urinating and from his own description, he was in one heck of a mess. He became acquainted with an old Hungarian woman who raised goats on a small farm near his home. He thought perhaps the goats' milk might help him so he made regular visits to her for this purpose. The lady loaned him a few books and suggested that he try natural foods. It was then that he first came to our establishment.

"There is no use denying it," he says, "at fifty-six I was an old man and felt it."

He began making the change in his eating and living habits according to information he found in the various books he read. His diet today consists of practically all raw food. His job is that of a day laborer. He works hard physically.

He was subjected to much kidding from his fellow

workers about the rabbit food he was eating. When they saw what he ate for lunch they would say, "You can't do a day's work on that bit of grass."

"It made me smile," he said. "I'd start to work with them in the morning. At ten o'clock they'd be puffing and be glad for the respite they would get during the coffee break. Of course, they'd have a cigarette. I didn't take the coffee break — I kept on working.

"At noon they'd sit down to their sandwiches and coffee and pies and cakes and I'd chew away at my vegetables and fruits. At five o'clock they were almost bow-legged and could hardly make it to their cars. I walked out as straight as a ramrod and then went home to prepare my own juices and salad. And they told me that the stuff I ate was only good for rabbits!"

Today he is in perfect health — no aches, no pains, no lumps, no bumps. He is active, robust, handsome and alert — a tribute to good living.

*George Roberts*

When I first knew this man his face had a distinct yellowish color and by no stretch of the imagination could he have been called a healthy looking individual. "But," he told me, "you should have seen me a year or two ago."

In those days he weighed 220 lbs. and more, smoked over a dozen cigars a day and drank with everybody and by himself. Then his health gave way and he ran from doctor to doctor but his condition grew worse.

One day he picked up some literature on the hygienic way of living and he thought it made sense, so he began to follow it.

When I met him three years ago he had effected many drastic changes in his life. He was thin — practically skin and bones — and he had that yellowish cast that I mentioned. Today he follows the rules almost with precision, eating practically only raw foods, with the exception of home-made soup.

The yellowish color is gone, his step is as lithe as that of a cat. I walked with him for a few miles on various occasions and I could hardly keep up with him. He is ten years older than I and I am considered a good walker by any standards.

Among other ailments which had assailed him, he claims that he got rid of an eye cataract with fasting and following the hygienic diet.

### Agnes Parsons

She used to come into the establishment every Saturday to pick up a few of our unsulphured fruits and some peanut butter. From what I could tell, this was about the only form of natural living that she practised. She didn't say very much but I gathered that she was not as well as she would have liked to be. She showed me on various occasions a sore on her face that didn't respond to any form of treatment and wouldn't heal.

She kept it well covered with make-up. Evidently this sore was the cause of her trying the natural foods. But I would have said that these foods would not have composed more than one-tenth of her diet.

When I returned from my travels in China, I heard that Agnes had a cancer of the cervix and had been given the bomb treatment. When she came in to see me a few days later I chatted with her and she told me about having the bomb treatment and that that was all they could do for her.

So I said, "Well, you've had the works. Now, how about trying natural living?"

She seemed to think it was a good idea so I suggested that she go down to one of the hygienic fasting institutions to learn how to live. I said, "I don't think they'll fast you because evidently fasting is not generally advised in cases where cancer is involved, but at least you can learn how to live and what to eat."

She said she would try it, but she didn't do very much about it.

About two months slipped by and she did write and get in touch with one of these organizations. But she told me she couldn't get away for family reasons and offered apologies and excuses.

Then, one day, much to my surprise, I received a note from her saying she was undergoing a fast. I was very much surprised at the turn of events. Evidently her condition had worsened. Otherwise, she would not have taken this drastic step.

She was gone four weeks and when I saw her she was much thinner but looked quite well. She was very much perturbed about the loss of weight and wanted to put it back on as quickly as possible.

Well, fifteen months have gone by. She still does not follow a rigid natural food or raw food diet but she is alive and I would say, comparatively well.

I try to reason with her and tell her she should go 100%. But so far I haven't been able to convince her. Nevertheless, she is active, attractive, pleasant and looks forward to many years of life.

Is she younger than she was two or three years ago? Well, of course you can answer that question yourself, considering she had been given up . . . a true terminal case. Today Agnes is more attractive and healthier than she has been in many years. She has not only grown younger . . . she's a new woman!

# CHAPTER 2

## Paving the Way

*"Too many people still believe in cures and in spite of my protest that I cannot cure anything, they come and assume the attitude; 'Here I am, now it is up to you to cure me.' They are foolish enough to believe that a cure should be made without any effort or any trouble on their part ... Living haphazardly, guessing how to live when dependable knowledge can be had, is a foolish and inexcusable hazard ... I repeat, I cannot cure, but I can teach all who crave knowledge, how to live to cure themselves and then how to live to stay well."*

; . . . J. H. TILDEN, M.D.

### NO SUBSTITUTE FOR KNOWLEDGE

Knowledge can make you rich, knowledge can make you free, knowledge can bring you health and long life.

With it you are a giant among men. Without it you're a pygmy. So come on, get cracking ... knowledge is available to you freely, just as it is to every other man in America if not in the world.

If you are sick, if you have troubles, if you have pain, if you are suffering, if you are poor, if you are unloved, if you are hated, if you are unpopular, knowledge can help you correct any or all of these conditions.

If you are poor, you can still gain knowledge because the finest literature in the world is free at the many thousands of public libraries throughout America.

You can take knowledge in small doses, in medium doses, in big doses or in mammoth doses. You can spend fifteen minutes a day acquiring knowledge or you can spend fifteen hours a day — revelling in it, steeping yourself in it, allowing it to permeate you through and through.

I have contended for many years that no one worthy of the name of man ought to permit the day to end without having learned something that he didn't know when that day began. It was the famed Doctor Eliot of Harvard who laid down the principle that fifteen minutes a day for ten years will give any ordinary man sufficient knowledge to earn a college degree. Therefore, you can readily see what an hour or two hours a day over a period of years can do.

I am not just spouting idle words for I have lived by that principle. It was Dr. Eliot who set for me my pattern of study.

However, I must stress that the selection of reading material is vitally important. It is admitted that you can waste your time by reading the wrong things. I am sorry to admit that I know many people, some of them close to me, who waste their lives in this way. But, in most cases, they are reading for relaxation and entertainment or escape (usually from themselves).

Do not allow yourself to believe it can't be done or permit yourself to think in the following channel . . . "How can I, in a short space of time, gain sufficient knowledge to benefit my health and improve my way of life, when doctors, healers and scientists have spent many years in college, practice and research and they can't do it?"

Well, let me tell you this. Most of the people who went to college spent the greater part of their time reading, studying and learning things that had little or no use or application in their later lives or even in their professions. They had no choice — and this is important — they had no choice in what they read and studied once they had set their path for a specific profession.

You, on the other hand, have the right of choice. If you want to study health, for example, you can learn all phases . . . the natural and the chemical. You can learn from the view of the scientist, the professor or the naturalist. You can also read the conservative, the radical, the reactionary and the old and the new. And your progress is limited only by your available time and your powers of perception.

So my advice to you is, *start now* Don't permit another day to go by without doing something to improve yourself mentally. It is clear that the mental is interwoven with the physical. So therefore, you will benefit your body, too, and you can be healthy and live to a ripe old age . . . of yes 70, 80, 90 and even 100. Why not? Others have done it before, and what one person has done, someone else can do better.

The obvious fact that with each passing year the scientific text books change — as they have been changing for centuries — is proof that the prescribed, accepted teaching in chemistry, pharmacology, medicine, surgery and other sciences of today in the universities is the lie of tomorrow.

But when we delve into the realm of nature and view her simple rules of living we see that her laws are as immutable today as they were 10,000 years ago and as they will be at the millennium.

## READING IS THE SOLUTION

No man need die prematurely of what we term natural causes if he possessed a bit of knowledge. Every man could extend his tenure of life if he had a little knowledge. No man need suffer ill health if he gains knowledge soon enough. No man need be stricken by disease if he has sufficient knowledge. It is the road to riches, to fame, to a better life, to health, to success, to greatness — yet so few avail themselves of the opportunity to acquire knowledge about the natural way of life. Why is it so?

I must admit that the pursuit of knowledge is time consuming. Most men, young or old, returning from a day's work, hard or light, find snoozing on the chesterfield or listening to the TV or sitting in a beer parlor guzzling beer, far more pleasurable than sitting hunched over a desk and poring over the printed word.

Knowledge is not come by easily or by merely wishing. It must be bought and paid for by toil (brain toil, I mean) and perhaps a strain upon the eyes . . . but the benefits are manifold and the effects far-reaching.

I don't care where your aims might lie or which field of endeavour you wish to select, knowledge will pay good dividends. The man I pity more than any man on earth — yes, even more than the man who is blind or ill — is the man who has never discovered the joy and potential of reading.

I could shed tears for those who have not learned the wonder, the beauty, the glory and the benefits that can be found in reading. I care very little about what they read, as long as they read.

Yes, I know there is poor literature, printed trash and good literature, but the average person, once he takes to reading, will know the good from the bad.

The greatest gift that a parent can pass on to his offspring is the joy, the pleasure, the enchantment that one gets from reading. There is no dividend or reward that I know of in life that even remotely compares with the wealth and riches that one derives from reading.

The time to read is when you are young, when your mind is most receptive and sponge-like ... ready, willing and eager to absorb. It is my belief that lessons learned in youth are indelible and are seldom if ever forgotten — whereas the lessons learned later in life seem to be more easily erasable.

So encourage the youth about you ... your children, your grandchildren, your nephews and nieces ... to read. And while you are doing that, put in a little time reading yourself. Set them a good example and absorb some genuine enlightenment and pleasure at one and the same time.

The giving of gifts has become a popular pastime in our present day world. I must commend this most civilized habit. Christians have the right idea and should lead the world in giving because did not Christ say, "It is more blessed to give than to receive?"

Now some people just like to give. It doesn't make any difference whether they give you a cigarette, an alcoholic drink, a new hat, or a bouquet of flowers. They enjoy, they revel in the sensation of giving. Perhaps they like to see the expression of surprise, pleasure or even gratitude upon the face of the recipient.

So it is to you who are the givers that I'm addressing this bit of writing. When you bestow why not give something that will be treasured, remembered and perhaps revered from the first moment until the last day? If you

27

give chocolates, candies, fruit, a bottle of cheer or some other tidbit, an hour or two after the gift has been received it is gone and forgotten.

This is all well and good, but you can do better — much better. For example, you might give something like perfume or flowers which last a few days or a few weeks . . . but it is still a case where the good deed, the noble thought, was there and now it is gone — and that is fine.

However, let us fly higher. My advice to you is that if you give something, give the finest in the world and let it take the form of a good book.

So, in the future when you are planning gifts for those about you, those you respect, admire and love, give them books and enhance their welfare.

## FOX AND GRAPES

Youth should be taught but never forced to accept any preconceived limited dogma.

Our conception of education — yes, throughout the Western world — is wrong, dead wrong. We teach our boys and girls to use the pedantic concept of knowledge and their talents to fashion things; to build empires, to create and fashion business enterprises; construct aeroplanes, dams, bridges; to build ships and U-boats. We do everything but guide them along the path that would make them true humanitarians or teach them to think for themselves or teach them how to live.

Nowhere along the path of my formal education, which was the same as yours and everyone else's, was I told that there is a reward for those of us who think and reason for ourselves . . . in fact, if you dare to think for yourself, you are slapped down and sat upon. Often for this bit of effrontery your scholastic career is abruptly brought to an end.

My English teacher in High School was a wonderful teacher . . . and she hated my guts because I would not accept the precepts, the concepts and the rules and laws that she laid down before me. You couldn't say "ain't" and you weren't allowed to split an infinitive; you were not allowed to use any of the four letter words that form the basis of our English language. If you'd use one of these good old basic Anglo-Saxon words, if it were up to her, you'd be flunked.

I argued with her and claimed there was only one language — the language that was spoken on the streets by the people — and no language ever rose above the level of the masses, no matter what she said

Some day we'll learn to encourage those who choose to think for themselves rather than brainwash them. We deride the Russians for their brainwashing techniques, yet we are every bit as bad in this respect, but we don't see the beam in our own eye.

It has been my experience that men with academic degrees and training cannot even comprehend how any man can think or negotiate or solve a problem without their specific kind of training . . . yet there are men in business and in other fields of endeavor who have reached great heights without that lofty training.

I have also known men who would not have been the men they were if they had had that training. Yes, often when I have investigated and read of men who reached the top rung of their fields by their bootstraps, I learned that at school they were poor students or barely made their passing grades.

I know what you're thinking — you're assuming I, too, was a lousy student; you're thinking that I didn't make my grades, and that is why I am espousing the cause of the individualist, the misfit, the down-trodden.

Well, even if it were true, I still maintain that mine is a point of view that deserves some consideration and if given a chance it will ultimately result in an improvement in our educational system. And by the name of all that we hold dear, it is high time that we made a change for the better.

You've heard of people dying from various causes . . . heart disease, pneumonia, cancer, asthma, spinal meningitis or any one of the hundred and one different things that people die from . . . but you've never heard of anyone dying from ignorance, have you?

But what if I were to tell you that 99 out of 100 untimely deaths are due to exactly that specific disease? Yes, I call it a disease because it is a disease. The only difference between ignorance and other diseases is that ignorance is self-inflicted. Of course the other diseases are basically that, too, I must admit . . . actually the end result of ignorance.

It has long been my belief that if you would cure ignorance, you would cure most of the diseases to which the human race is subject. Please believe me when I tell you that I, too, almost perished from that selfsame disease — ignorance!

When people tried to guide me so that I would cure my ignorance, I laughed at them — I derided them — I even insulted them. That just proves how profound and deeply ingrained was my ignorance. But some of them perhaps thought that I was worth saving and persisted and came back at me. Eventually I saw the light . . . but not because they showed it to me and led me there, but because a few little things began to go wrong and I sensed the thin end of the wedge and began to do a bit of investigating on my own.

That is why today I try my level best to help cure the disease of ignorance in others . . . because knowledge is the positive cure for that and other diseases. My favorite cry to people is "Read this" or "Read that" . . . "Investigate" . . . "Make comparisons and do a little thinking."

Nobody is forcing you to do anything or accept anything, but please, you owe it to yourself to investigate. When I think of how I scoffed at people who tried to tell me that raw food was the answer! Well, the simple truth was that I enjoyed filling my belly with those delectable cooked and processed viands. But when at last I realized that I had a choice between disease and untimely death with conventional food and good health with raw food, there was no hesitation and I made the choice. And I am glad ... even though I do miss my hotdog and my hamburg, my bacon and eggs, my French fries, my coffee and cookies and cakes and pies.

Yes, I outwardly admit that I miss them ... but I would never go back to them for all the rice in China, for all the wheat in Canada or for all the gold in Fort Knox.

## MAN'S GREATEST ENEMY

I don't know whether or not you have found this true in your lifetime but I have found that my greatest enemy is myself. I can usually get by in dealing with my fellow man ... I am the boy I've got to worry about mainly.

In going over my life in retrospect and looking at it with a clear understanding attitude, I am quite convinced that practically all of the grief and troubles and worries that I have found along the way were caused by one person and that person was John H. Tobe. My lifetime of observation and experience has taught me that this holds true for you just as much as it does for me and for all other human beings.

Sure, you can blame others for your plight or your poverty or your lack of opportunity but when you get it down to cold, naked truths, you'll find that the man to blame for the fact that you didn't get where you had hoped to get and where you wanted to get was ... you. I ask you to study the matter yourself, be fair and honest, and you can't reach any other conclusion.

Oh, I surely do recognize the truth that no man likes to blame himself. Sure, 99 people out of 100 prefer to blame someone else ... wives blame their husbands, husbands blame their wives, children blame their parents, parents blame their children, brother blames sister, sister blames brother, friend blames friend and friend blames enemy ... and this goes on endlessly.

31

But if you don't get on in life, if you don't become a success or if you don't make friends, it is your fault!

By the same token, the biggest obstacle in your path towards good health and long life is that stumbling block known as *you*! So the man you've got to deal with in order to accomplish this goal is yourself.

Well, right here and now I'll say this to you. It is your habits that are causing your trouble — whether it's eating habits, sleeping habits, drinking habits, sexual habits, social habits, working habits or any one of a hundred and one other habits to which a human being is addicted. These are your enemies and before you can get anywhere you must conquer them.

For instance, you might have the habit of drinking tea or coffee. Before you can enjoy perfect health or even strive for good health, you're going to have to break that habit. You might like very hot soup or beverages or other hot foods. Well, before you're going to get anywhere noticeably, you're going to have to break that habit. Then you may like ice cream, you may like French fries and you may like any one of a thousand other things that are definitely harmful. I can do nothing for you — you must do this for yourself.

I probably like most of the things you like and dislike the things you dislike. I like wine, I like song, I like girls— young and old — I like pleasures, I like fun. Anything you like, I like too. But above all, I like living and I want to go on living as long as I can and in the best health that I can command.

I had to break the habit of using salt, of using lots of condiments, of eating mostly cooked foods, of eating smoked, pickled and fresh meat and fish, of drinking beer and wine, of smoking, of eating big meals of highly seasoned, wonderful tasting, glorious cooked foods and I had to give up partying and weekending. Do I need to go on? I had to give up 99 out of 100 things that I loved.

Well, you can say right here and now, "To hell with it! If I've got to give up all those things, I don't want it!" But let me tell you this. I've seldom known a man, when he was sick, ailing or dying, who wouldn't gladly give up all of those things if he could have a few more months or a few more years of precious life.

I am reminding you of this very forcibly because I saw it happen to one of my own kith and kin. It was all right for him to shout, "Oh, to hell with it! If I've got to give up all the things I enjoy, who wants life?" Yet when this selfsame person was stricken, he cried, "O Lord, why did you afflict me thus?" and he wrung his hands and wept copious, bitter tears. This is the usual pattern.

Then, too, you and you alone have to decide whether or not ten or twenty five years of added life make it worthwhile giving up most of these contemptible things that you have learned to like, love and enjoy. First of all, let me assure you that you are not giving up anything ... you are just shaking leeches from your body that have clung to you since infancy.

This I'll concede ... the bad habits to which you fell heir were positively not your fault. They were the gift of civilization. Or should I say that your mother or your father gave them to you? From the moment they gave you a bottle — that is, a bottle with a nipple at the end, filled with cow's milk or milk and water or sugar and water — they addicted you to a very bad habit. Then from there you went to cooked foods, for they thought that a baby couldn't eat or digest raw foods ... and from that day onward you were in trouble.

Therefore, all of these habits were presented to you as gifts. If they had started you off by feeding you good, wholesome, natural fruits and vegetables and nuts, you would have learned to love proper food and there would be no need to break these insidious habits. But that is not the way it happens in this world. Man has never risen to those heights of intelligence — to follow the proper way of living.

So in reality you're not giving up anything — you're just getting back to where you should have been in the first place. These things that you think you like or look upon as good are mainly contemptibles which continued use taught you to like.

33

When I gave up salt, the world just about ended for me right then and there. For six months I seldom enjoyed a mouthful of food. I think I hated myself and everybody else. I was a sour, miserable man. But I had said I'd never use a salt shaker again as long as I lived and I meant it. I had learned that salt was my enemy and I was through with it!

Then because I saw signs of degeneration appearing in my body, I wanted to switch to whole, natural, raw foods as rapidly and as painlessly as possible. Oh, it was tough! Here is the way I worked it out with myself. I resolved to go on a strictly vegetable or fruit diet once a week — that is, all raw. I looked forward to the day with dread ... but as soon as I was into that day, I was looking forward to the next day when I could go back to eating the things I wanted to eat. And from that stunt I progressed slowly but surely.

I recognized first the great value of those one-day-a-week raw food binges. Then I tried it for two days a week ... then alternate days ... and the benefits seemed to pile up. Now I only allow myself some cooked food for one meal a day and I'm as happy as a lark about it.

I swear that I haven't aged a day since I became almost a complete raw-fooder. I honestly believe, from what I see and hear, that I appear younger in every way than I did when I started this stunt.

I have known people who have made the transition by going on a fast, for ten days or thirty days or more, and when they finished their fast, they switched over to the new hygienic way of life. However, the method of conversion rests entirely upon yourself. You know your own limitations, you know your own strength of character and therefore, you have to figure out a plan of attack that will suit you.

## I MAKE MY CHOICE

Many of my friends have taken issue with me frequently concerning my faith in empiricism rather than in science.

If tomorrow a situation arose on which my life depended and before me I had evidence from empirical sources that showed one thing and evidence from scientific sources showed another, even at the risk of my life I would accept the empirical proof.

I reason it this way. The scientist in reaching his conclusion might have made a mistake. The scientist in reaching his conclusion accepted the findings of one, two or many researchers before him. He also accepted the mathematical and scientific equations that he was taught, yet which were not always proven in practice. Scientists do make mistakes, you know. For example, where have all of those wonderful scientific discoveries in drugs of yesteryear gone?

Then I lay before you the case of the empiricist.

For 3,000 or more years they have found that a poultice of bread and milk will relieve swellings or cause draining of suppurating sores. They do not know why, but they do know that it brings the desired result. This is but a simple example of empiricism versus science at work.

You have a right to follow the path that you deem best.

# CHAPTER 3

## Sick America

*The soft life has a serious sting in it. The effects of it are making themselves evident in the type of illness to which we fall heir. Primitive natives claim a higher degree of health and freedom from mental and physical illness than we with our civilized softness.*

... J. DeWITT FOX, M.D.

### PERILOUS, PRECARIOUS

I'm confronted with a dilemma — a serious dilemma — one that is causing me a great deal of grief and heartache.

"What is your dilemma?" you ask. Well, one part of me says, "Buy yourself a little farm somewhere, Tobe, in the back woods and settle down, do a little work, do a little writing, do a little thinking and let the rest of the world go by."

Man, oh man, that's what I want to do. Every fibre in my heart and soul says, "Go do it. That's what you've wanted. That's what you've dreamed about. That's what you've longed for."

And that's true. You may not believe me but I have never wanted to be a millionaire or even a rich man. I don't want fame and I don't want a fortune. But I do want and do seek the respect of my fellow man.

Sometimes I don't know whether I'm accursed or blessed, but through the past few years a vast amount of knowledge concerning health and nutrition has come my way. Then I realize that most of the ills of mankind are precisely due to the lack of this knowledge. So what am I to do? Ignore it? Keep this knowledge to myself?

While most of mankind is lacking in this vital knowledge, there is a greater evil astir. Unbeknown to most people, practically all of our food is being so treated, adulterated, changed and processed as to render it unfit for human or animal use. Not only is it unfit for use, it is harmful, it is deadly. The simple, bold, plain, unadulterated

36

truth is that we are positively being poisoned by every mouthful of food that we put into our bodies.

I want to warn you. The situation is so alarming that I believe that 90% of all deaths, apart from accidents, are caused by the poisons in our foods ... and that goes for the simplest commodities in our diet like sugar, bread margarine, jam, cheese or meat. I doubt if there is a packaged or processed commodity that you can buy in any store in America that does not contain chemical additives that are harmful or deadly.

Yes, this extends to your jar of peanut butter or your soup mixes or your cake mixes or the meat that you buy at your butcher's or even the dried fruit that you buy. Yes, they are all treated with harmful, murderous chemicals. "But," you say, "our government does not permit such things to happen." And I tell you this ... that there is no such thing as a harmless chemical put into your food. Each and every one does you harm.

The illnesses that you suffer from today are caused by the food that you ate a year ago, two years ago and even ten years ago. Please don't laugh and think that I'm joking or that I've gone berserk. I swear to you that every statement I make can be attested to by irrefutable documented clinical proof. So I ask you not to take this lying down. Inquire, dig, find out and don't allow yourself to be tranquilized and slowly dinned to death to the tune of fancy phrases like, "We are the best fed people in the world. We have the finest supply of wholesome food in the world."

The truth is that America today is one of, if not *the* sickest nation on the face of the earth and will be a lot sicker in the days immediately following. Please believe me, I am not a blues singer or a calamity caller. I speak the truth.

The situation is much worse, much more tragic than any words that I can use or any warning that I can echo.

## BIGGEST NOT BEST

When someone, no matter who it is, tells you that we are

the healthiest people in the world, that we have the best food supply in the world, that we have the best balanced diet in the world and that we in America are living longer than ever before, ask him for proof!

Tell him to produce the statistics or shut up!

Now the only proof that he'll be able to offer is that America produces the most food . . . and it does. America has the best farm equipment in the world by far — so superior to the rest of the world that it isn't even comparable — and that has given America a tremendous supply of food. It is not the best food nor the most nutritious, but I agree that it is the most abundant. It could be the most nutritious and it could be the best food, if it were grown in the old fashioned way, except for using mechanized equipment which is a credit to American ingenuity.

Don't let anyone tell you that we now have a higher life expectancy than ever before for that is nothing but a blatant lie and the figures offered by the United States Government prove that it is a lie. Furthermore, you don't have to go very far to prove it to yourself. Read the obituary column in your daily paper and see the ages of those who are dying. Then get the mortality statistics that are available from many sources. You will see, you will be appalled at the tremendous number of people who die in youth or early in middle life.

I predict that soon, very soon, you and most of us will learn that we cannot trust anyone with our foods. Therefore, there will be no other course to follow but to "grow your own" . . . which will mean that America will once more become an agricultural nation!

If we are to survive, that is the path of survival. No, I am in dead earnest — I'm not joking. Nor am I day-dreaming. It is fast becoming clear that those of us who want to live and retain our health will see the light and find our way onto a farm.

It won't have to be a big farm. In fact, we'll find that it is most sensible and economical to have a farm where we can be completely self-sustaining.

Soon those who live in the cities will recognize the truth

of what I say and they will also know that there is no alternative. If they are to survive they must grow their own food.

Therefore, I predict a tremendous "back to the land" movement. And you know what? I'm going to be among the first to head in that direction.

## GREAT, RICH, WONDERFUL — BUT

It is true that America is the richest country in the world. It is true that America has the greatest food supply of any country in the world. It is true that America has more automobiles than any country in the world ... and more telephones, better clothing, more drugs, more physicians, more surgeons. Oh, I could go on and the list would be endless. It is clear that America has more material things than any country on the face of the earth.

Yes, and it is also true that America has the greatest number of scientists and the greatest scientists in the world. Yes, and with all the great amount of knowledge disseminated by our great universities and higher schools of learning, still cancer is rotting out our civilization. You see, in spite of all the wonderful things that America can do, they cannot positively cure cancer.

Even with the hundreds of millions of dollars collected and spent for cancer and heart disease, they cannot cure it. I suggest we have drifted from the path of sane, common, logical thinking. What good is our wealth and our civilization, our material things and our science? I will let you answer this question for yourself.

## SICKNESS IS BIG BUSINESS

I am the most unloved person in the world.

No, I'm not feeling terribly sorry for myself. I'm a unique case ... I thrive on being unloved.

How could I expect people to love me? I seek to put the chemical people out of business. I seek to do away with the drug manufacturers. I claim there is no need for healers. I say that there should be no need for hospitals. I suggest that food processors harm the food we eat. I would take the bread out of the mouths of hundreds of thousands of people.

Neither you nor I nor anyone can deny that sickness with its involvements is today the biggest and most thriving industry in America.

Sure, we need healers and many more than we have today . . . because we are not getting any healthier, we are getting sicker . . . and healers are required to help us along in this great economic pursuit of health. Yes, I said pursuit . . . but we'll never catch up, because health can't be found via the pursuit system. You don't hunt health with bloodhounds. You don't hunt it with a snare and a trap. You don't hunt it with lures. Health can be found in only one way — through correct direction by means of enlightenment and through natural living and proper diet.

So because I would take the bread from the mouths of millions, no one sings my praises.


## WHAT IS A HOTDOG?

America, the land of the brave and the free

Well, I contend we're not free and I know we're no longer brave. If we were, we wouldn't be putting up with what we are.

I don't know where the word "hamburg" originated . . . or "hotdog" or "French fries" or "ice cream" or "ketch-up" . . . but when I knew these things 40 or 50 years ago, a hamburg was ground up meat fried on a griddle, stashed between two hunks of bread or a bun and it cost a nickel. A hotdog was sort of a weiner — plain ground up meat that was mostly beef — put up in a covering of skin from the guts of an animal. Then it was cooked, pressed into a bun, smeared with mustard and that was it. French fries were cut up strips of potatoes dipped into boiling fat. Ice cream was cream and sugar, eggs, fruit flavoring and perhaps nuts.

Those were the names that the American public gave these commodities and in the good old days that's what you paid for and that's what you got. Now by what right, by what authority, does the Food and Drug Administration connive with the processors to turn these foods into horrible chemical concoctions?

Do you know what a hamburg is today? Let me tell you. Pulverized meat from a hog, sheep or cow, water, salt, sugar, ascorbic acid, sodium nitrate, sodium nitrite hydrolized vegetable protein, artificial flavoring, diethylstilbestrol. Do you know what a hotdog is today? It's all the things a hamburg is, plus a cellophane-type wrapping, plus horrible chemical dyes and chemical seasonings, plus filling agents.

Do you know what ice cream is? It's a whole batch of synthetic chemicals sometimes containing cream. And French fries . . . a detergent-covered, dip-treated potato dipped into a concoction that is worse than axle grease or motor oil.

These things that I have mentioned to you are all done with the permission and the assent of the Food and Drug Administration . . . and then they tell you that you are being protected. What they don't tell you is that it is not you who are being protected — it is the processor and the chemical corporations that are protected. You, the consumer, are being hornswoggled!

## SAFE, SURE INVESTMENT

If you have money to invest and are looking for the best investment, I would advise you to buy chemical fertilizer stock and any stocks dealing with sickness, for today sickness is the biggest business in America, if not in the world.

Let me show you how sure and safe is the investment in the chemical business. To begin with, the chemical boys sell you chemical fertilizers because they have figures to prove that it will get more out of your soil. Then after five or ten years of robbing and throwing your soil out of balance, your plants begin to get sick because of the forcing and the effects of the chemical poisoning. So then you get bugs and disease and fungus and virus and everything else. Then the

41

experimental stations and agricultural representatives advise cures ... and the chemical companies' salesmen come along and they sell you chemicals (to treat the conditions that the other chemicals brought about) in the form of sprays, dusts, fungicides, insecticides and other searing, life-destroying concoctions. And of course, the people who eat the plants from these impoverished soils get sick too ... so then they sell them antibiotics and drugs to try to make them well again — or at least mask the symptoms.

So there you have it! Everybody is affected by these chemicals ... the soil, the micro-organisms, the plants, the animals that eat the plants and then the humans that eat the plants and animals. So they get you from the cradle to the grave, they get you from the soil to the body. It is unqualifiedly the most beautiful scheme that was ever brought to earth. What a nefarious occupation ... but if you're interested in making money, you'll buy their stocks.

If you can't lick 'em, join 'em. It is without doubt the world's best business and will soon be, if it is not already the world's biggest business!


## PREVENTION BETTER THAN TEARS

There sits before me a report contending that the U.S. infant death rate is too high. This statement was made by a March of Dimes physician. It shows that 25.3 children under one year die per 1,000 births in the United States and 27.2 in Canada.

This article goes on to blame the fact that the young mothers did not report to the prenatal clinics for advice.

Well, let me say this. Perhaps if they went to the clinics for prenatal advice, it would help, but I think the answer lies in an entirely different direction. If these young women and mothers would stop heeding the advice they get over the television and radio and in their magazines and from the government agencies, they would, in my humble opinion, give birth to healthier children and the infant death rate would drop.

No mention is made of the grave dangers in cigarette

smoking and drinking, be it beer, cocktails, coffee or pop.

You don't have to go very far for the true reason for the high infant mortality rate. Right here we also have the cause and reason why millions of children are born with various congenital defects. If the mothers before and during pregnancy were fed decent, wholesome, natural foods and were given no drugs and they did not have chemicals forced upon them in practically every food they ate, then they would give birth to healthy children and the infant mortality rate would sink to a low, low level.

I think it is the duty of every parent or grandparent or sane-thinking individual to warn young married women of the dangers in smoking, in drinking beer and liquor, in tranquilizers and other drugs, as well as lots of coffee and cold drinks.

It is better to take these precautions than to have the heartbreak of having a stillborn child or having the child die before it is a year old or having to raise a retarded, palsied, deformed or crippled child.

If the above precautions were taken, the mothers and fathers would then have little cause for regret.

Please pass this information on to all would-be mothers and others who will listen.

# CHAPTER 4

## Nature's Path

*Depleted soils produce deficient foods and deficient foods bring us ill health ... . Two food items may look alike, but one may have everything such a food should have because it was grown on healthy soil while the other is worth no more than a glass of water if grown on sick soil.*

§ § § § DR. WM. A. ALBRECHT

## THE NATURAL WAY OF LIFE

A half century of living, observing, contemplating, and studying along with what little intuition I still retain have clearly demonstrated to me that the natural way of life is the best.

It is best because it will enable a man to remain in good health and live longer than any other known way of life. But following the natural way of life does not necessarily mean that we must resort to primitive customs and ways of living.

Even with the small variety of vegetables cultivated in our society, most people still remain unacquainted with many of the vegetables and fruits available at the better food markets; for example, egg plant, zucchini squash, endive, broccoli, papaya, mango and others. I have put this matter to a test frequently by asking people to name different kinds of vegetables that can be used in a fresh salad. I learn that few can name beyond five ... lettuce, celery, cucumber, radish and tomato ... whereas there are at least forty kinds available every single day in the better food markets.

My travels have clearly indicated that the primitive way of life is not necessarily the proper or the best way of life and it should not be confused with the natural way of life. What I advocate is following the teachings of nature but doing so only after careful study, close scrutiny, practice and research.

44

You may be tempted to ask, "Why is the primitive way of life not the proper way of life?"

My answer to that question requires a bit of explanation. Somewhere back many thousands of years when man first learned how to control fire, he also learned how to cook his food and since that day he has believed that cooking improves the nutritional quality of his food. Even the most primitive people on earth cook their food. Today, many people, like the Chinese and the Indians, feel that no food is fit to eat unless it is cooked.

My studies and investigations reveal clearly that the widespread practice of cooking is one of man's gravest errors. He has clung to that erroneous belief and faulty way of life for thousands of years — to his detriment, for it has shortened his span of life drastically.

I have found that nowhere else on earth do people use as much raw food as we do in America. Oh yes, I realize that we do far too much cooking too, yet our consumption of raw food far exceeds that of any other country. I might even go further and say that we use more raw foods in America than all the rest of the world together.

From close on-the-scene observations in Abyssinia, Borneo, the Philippine Islands, China, Japan, India, Pakistan, Afghanistan and thirty or more other countries, ranging from the primitive to very old civilizations, I have reached the conclusion that we here in America have a greater knowledge of the proper way of life than do most other peoples on earth.

There are more books and more guides on proper living in America than are to be found in any other part of the world . . . but by the same measure, there are more books on the incorrect, on the false, on the detrimental way of life published in America than in any other country in the world.

So the big and important question is, "How can one tell the true doctrine from the false doctrine?"

My suggestion is to read both sides and then make your decision. If you think that man is wiser than nature, then you'll have to side with the chemical and the additive and the chemical fertilizer and the synthetic way of living. On the other hand, if you believe that nature knows best, then is it not wise and sensible to follow in the ways of natural living?

I believe that every man, every family should have their own garden where they can grow part of their food supply. A plot of ground builds character in people, especially children. It gives one a sense of security, enables families to work together, play together and live together and enjoy the fruits of their labors and have good wholesome food. Of course, it is a big money-saver, besides.

Living in the city permits a man too much leisure. What with working only seven or eight hours a day five days a week, with many holidays, a man definitely does not get enough exercise. Besides, there are very few vocations or positions in our society today that enable a man to perform much physical labor. With the exception of stevedoring, truck driving, warehousing and some few other labor-expending jobs, physical labor is a thing of the past. This is one of the prices one must pay for the privilege of the city life.

Further, in the city there is an extensive amount of smog or factory smoke or dust and dirt and what is much worse, gasoline fumes . . . all of which are now part and parcel of city living. In some quarters they claim that the fumes in the city are as much a contributor to lung cancer as smoking.

It must also be taken into consideration that TV watching is not a healthy pursuit. Apart from the fact that it keeps people seated for many hours every day, which is positively detrimental to health, the rays given off by the television set are considered by some authorities to be seriously harmful. Pregnant women are warned that television might be a factor in the rising number of cases of leukemia because the rays affect the unborn infant. My advice is not to ignore the warning of the dangers in TV viewing.

Even in a city one can still follow the natural way of life to a satisfactory degree . . . by eating natural foods, by getting enough exercise, by taking long walks in the parks where one can get good air, and by procuring by some means wholesome drinking water that has been neither chlorinated nor fluoridated.

Often I am asked, "Is the chlorination of our water supply necessary?"

After much thought and deep consideration, I have reached the following conclusion. Where people desire to live like bees in hives, one on top of another, then the treating of the drinking water supply with bacteria-destroying drugs (of which chlorine is but one) may be warranted. But lest you or anyone else be misled, please understand that by this selfsame treatment many protective and beneficial bacteria are also destroyed. Let us also remember that due to our wide use of alcoholic beverages, cigarettes and bacteria-destroying drugs, our gastro-intestinal bacterial flora are at a minimum or altogether destroyed and any unusual micro-organism in the water might induce varying degrees of sickness or disease. Thus the chlorination of water may be justified.

Good health is seldom an accident. It is not a gift from the gods — it requires many things, and understanding is not the least among them. The natural way of life implies healthful eating habits, healthful living habits and a healthful mental attitude. And we must never allow ourselves to forget the most vital consideration of all ... knowledge concerning food and health.

To those "who know it not" the natural way of life is but a phrase. Only a man who has suffered serious illness and pain and then found his way back to abundant health through the natural way of life can appreciate its true value.


## LETTER TO THE CHEMICAL INDUSTRY

The handwriting is on the wall — there is but little time left for stock taking or recriminations. This is in truth a letter, an appeal or perhaps a plea to the manufacturers of chemicals and drugs and all others occupied in these nefarious occupations and allied trades.

I would like to say to them, "Read this, please. It may

47

mean your own salvation as well as that of countless millions of innocent people."

Before you write me off as being completely out of my mind, think, ponder, look out, beware and listen a little longer.

The deviltry you are creating in our soil, our good mother earth, the violent imbalance you are causing, the eternal destruction of our vital enzymes, micro-organisms, bacteria, plant insects and other earth denizens is already becoming evident! But soon it will be even clearer.

I know that right now even as I write this article, you are having considerable trouble with varying crops in different widely scattered parts of the world where agriculture is being conducted as you like and advocate it, along strict chemical technical lines.

You are still blaming it on insects, bad management or covering it up in technical abracadabra — but you won't be able to keep using these old dodges very much longer because instead of these things occurring occasionally they will be so widespread that there will be no evasion of the truth. Soon you will find that most of the chemically treated crops that grow in our fields will never reach their destination in a condition fit to eat. Apart from the fact that they are loaded with chemicals and weren't fit to eat in the first place, they will rot or be absolutely unusable by man or beast before they reach the market.

I have seen with my own eyes many examples of this already. While most of those who saw this condition blamed it on frost, mishandling, unfavorable weather or various blights, or any one of a dozen different conditions, I knew and so did you, what the real trouble was.

Now you won't be able to fool yourself or the people throughout the country very much longer because it will be so obvious and so clear, that there will be no possibility of placing the blame elsewhere — as you have done for almost a hundred years.

Nature is starting to hit back. She is doing it already, and you, Mr. Chemical Fertilizer and Mr. Drug Manufacturer and Mr. Food Processor, are sitting on a powder keg of your own asking, filled with explosive chemicals that you made for other purposes . . . but you are going to be blown up along with them!

We have all read the reports of the fish dying in our lakes and rivers. However, on January 21, 1965, the shore along the Niagara River, was piled with millions of dead fish. And strewn among the fish were sea gulls — which indicates that the fish were deadly to anyone or anything that ate them.

## BE NATURAL

Life need not, should not end at seventy. The fact that men live to be 80 and 90 and even 100 and beyond is ample proof that it can be done. What one man has done another man can do better.

The big trouble as I see it is that when we should be learning and studying how to live, we are busy chasing up hill and down dale, down super-speed highways, across busy intersections . . . to snare a smoke, to snatch a drink, or grab a buck. Then when we get tripped up in this hectic procedure and land flat on our faces, we gaze about us bewildered and say, "What happened?"

Well, it's simply that you ran afoul of your own follies. Ah, but who can condemn you — that's the way it is with youth. And who am I to stay your hand or draw in the reins? I was once like that, too, and I didn't like the idea of a bit cutting into my mouth!

"It's my life, isn't it? I can do what I like with it. And if I want to throw it away, it's none of your business."

Yes, that's what you say when you're in your twenties. But when you're in your late thirties or forties, and double-trouble tracks you down, you say, "Why didn't someone tell me? Why didn't someone show me the error of my ways?"

The truth is they did try but your ears were stuffed with your egotism. You believed in the infallibility of youthful energy and wisdom.

49

It is true that man does not die before his time. If he succumbs, it is because he has killed himself.

A gun and a noose aren't the only means by which men reach their untimely end. A man can commit suicide by the food that he eats ... misguided by his ignorance.

You know as well as I do that if you plead ignorance when you have broken a law, it will not get you off or minimize your punishment. And by the same token, when your health breaks down and you plead ignorance, it will not help redeem your health ... unless you do something tangible about it while there is still time.

What to me is even a greater tragedy is the fact that so many people have the erroneous idea that to eat the proper foods, to follow a sensible, balanced diet, is akin to being sentenced to solitary confinement in a dungeon.

I have found that most dislikes, whether they be of people, food or drink, are usually based on ignorance. When enlightenment comes to a man's mind, he doesn't spend so much time disliking and hating.

We sometimes dislike who we don't know. When you get to know them better, you usually learn to like them or love them. The same applies to foods ... especially the natural foods that know no polish or primping.

A good man or woman doesn't need to be disguised. All of the truly beautiful women that I have known were beautiful before a bit of lipstick or rouge ever touched their luscious lips and cheeks. Their eyes were gleaming before the mascara and the eyebrow pencil ever besmirched them.

Well, that's the way I like women and food — simple, natural, uncontaminated. Learn to appreciate and love the natural foods. Sure, they need a little more thought and understanding ... but believe me, they're worth it!

## REFINED IS MALIGNED

When I was a youngster I believed and was given to understand that anything that was refined was improved or better. They spoke of refined foods, refined girls, refined culture. You know it took me half a century to realize that refinement was another word for contemptible. Nowadays when I hear the word "refined" I look for the thin edge of the wedge.

I understand they are making refined bullets now . . . so when they strike you, they'll go through the heart faster and perform the function of killing you more neatly and it won't leave an ugly hole in your body.

Refined foods and oils mean that every decent bit of value is removed from them and that all the coarseness has been eliminated and that it is silky smooth in texture . . . but otherwise useless.

This goes for all of these things: refined sugar, refined salt, refined oil, refined cereal grains.

One thing I've noticed for certain, too, is that they have also refined the way of giving you the works. Nowadays they give it to you so you don't even know you're getting it.

## NOT ONE BUT MANY

I have a confession to make. I have to admit that there is no such thing as a health food.

In our eagerness to help ourselves or to help others, we often label a food "a health food". It has been done by many people and I, too, have been guilty of that error . . . among the many other errors that I have committed.

I am of the opinion that no one single article of food can in itself be a guarantee of health. It is probably correct that some foods are better than others, but I think it would be better for all of us if we understood and accepted the fact that there is no one single food that will create health.

I also suggest that those of us who seek help and guidance and long life from foods refer to them as natural foods because therein lies health and long life.

It is becoming increasingly obvious that only natural foods can provide proper nutrition. The chemists, the drug manufacturers and even nutritionists can brag all they like about fortifiers, enriching agents and other such chemicals, but no means or method or process has ever been devised that can improve upon the natural goodness contained in nature's foods. I challenge any man on earth to refute that direct statement.

All good natural foods are health foods in that they provide nourishment and the nutrients required by the body to build and sustain good health. But to segregate them and say that any one or any group of foods is particularly a health food is erroneous.

Yes, there are many people — thousands, if not tens of thousands — who will attest to the fact that they have found benefits through yogurt, blackstrap molasses, brewer's yeast, alfalfa, soya beans, sunflower seeds, sesame seeds and many others ... but they are only part of the great variety of natural foods required by the human body.

I wish to go on record as stating that natural foods grown on good natural soil will provide health and well-being to the human body and yes, give long life, too. But you need a wide variety from nature's vast stock of provisions. Please, don't allow yourself to be fooled or misled into thinking that any one food will provide you with health or that it will cure any disease, sickness or ailment.

## WHICH IS WHICH?

Did you ever hear of the "mugwump" system of gardening?

This is the fellow we all know who sits on the garden fence and his "mug" is with the chemical boys and his "wump" is with the organic gang.

He's afraid to say that he uses manure because his friends and neighbors might shun him or have their noses twitch every time they see him approach.

Yet he doesn't trust chemicals and actually has a comparatively good organic garden. However, he takes no chances on pests, bugs and germs and he doesn't completely trust the organic system either, so he sprays and douses his plants with various insecticides and pesticides.

He doesn't even wait until they're attacked before he goes out on the rampage.

This "mugwump" system of his, spoils the good work he has done in raising organically grown produce by covering it with lethal doses of harmful, deadly sprays. So for appearance's sake he runs a bit with the hares and then he joins the hounds for the foray.

In truth I can't blame Mr. Mugwump because anyone who professes following even a branch of the natural way of living or gardening or farming is subject to ridicule and is the target of jests and jokes.

Really, it takes a brave man to stand and pit himself against the present day conventional gardeners.

No one can deny that it's no cinch to stand up and be counted and be on your guard at all times.

So I'll say this. We forgive you, Mr. Mugwump. Perhaps some day your convictions will be strengthened and you will, without fear or trepidation, join our ranks. And you know what? When you come to us, we'll look out for you as best we can and we'll also help to fortify you with the required intestinal fortitude to stand up against any and all attacks. Knowledge will make you free.


## NATURE DOES NOT FAIL

The older I get, the more I become convinced that good health is the right and just dessert of every mortal. But as you can clearly understand and have found out, we don't always get our just rights. They are sometimes denied us for any one of many reasons. In fact, most of us are indeed lucky that we do not get our due and just rights.

But this is what I want to say and I want to say emphatically. Good health is easy — yes, easy — because it's natural . . . and if natural, it is simple!

Whether you wish to gain, maintain or regain sound mental and bodily health, the way to do it is to follow the laws and the rules of nature. It always brings results, it can't fail to bring results — otherwise mankind would have perished from this earth a long, long time ago.

53

Provided with natural, balanced nourishment, the human body can take care of every challenge that besets it, whether from outside or from within.

It has been truly stated by many wise men that nature knows no incurable diseases — everything will respond to nature. Surely you can understand that a drug and chemical ridden body is not conforming to the laws or rules of nature and therefore nature is being frustrated and prevented from performing its proper, natural function.

So, I repeat that nature knows no incurable disease. Therefore, govern yourself accordingly!

## LUCKY OLD TIMERS

Would you believe me if I said that you and I who are comparative oldsters (anything over 40) have a great advantage over those younger folks, born and raised since the 30's? You may be one of those so-called unlucky ones who hasn't had it so good, perhaps due to the economy, but I'm still telling you that our way of life in those days was much better than the life they are leading today.

Sure, they have big shiny cars, slicker clothes and haberdashery, more entertainment, cockier cocktails and they eat fancier foods. But does all that compensate for the many vital human things that they are missing?

I was brought up rough, tough and ready, without any pampering ... but I did have a father and mother who were close by during all hours, day and night, and if I were missing for a few hours, they would want to know where and why.

Take the situation today — especially when so many mothers are working. From early morning till evening a mother never sees her child or the child never sees its mother. Is that good?

My mother was home from the time I got up in the morning until I went to bed at night. She watched everything I ate ... in fact, she prepared practically every mouthful. Now don't get any fancy ideas that I was a spoiled brat, an only child in the family, because there were nine of us kids. But Mom generally knew where all nine of us were during the day and night, too ... or else!

Today I don't think the mothers know or care too much where one or two are — probably because the service clubs, recreation centres, community groups or welfare organizations, including churches, provide systemized entertainment and some sort of care. Kids everywhere are raised with a sort of umbrella over them so they won't get wet, overheated, undernourished or strained.

I used to walk from Adelaide Street in Toronto to College Street on University Avenue to go to school — yes, spring, fall and winter. Four times a day I did this and I didn't even have rubbers or an overcoat to protect me from the wind, rain, snow, sleet, slush and those demoniacal icy blasts that howled down University Avenue. No, there was no bus to pick me up and cart me comfortably to my destination. I would judge that the trip to school was a bit less than two miles each way.

I skated on Toronto Bay and ice-boated when I could sneak or cajole a ride, and swam at the foot of John Street where the grain elevators are now located. There is no longer any incentive for individual initiative among youngsters ... no inner compulsion, no reason for get up and go, no striving from within to do things on their own.

In our house, when mother cooked soup, everybody drank soup. When mother served liver, everybody ate liver. When mom served grits, everybody grated grits. And not in my childhood and early youth do I recall one instance when one of us dreamt of saying we didn't like it or didn't want it. Why? ... Because there simply wasn't anything else. When we were growing boys and girls, the old kettle of soup (bones, meat and fat scrapings, and grains and vegetables) would sit on the stove and simmer. It was big enough for a child to bathe in — almost like a cannibal's stew pot — and we needed it that big too. Then, whatever part of the beef carcass was served, or the mutton for that matter, that was what we ate and that was what we liked.

The only complaint ever heard at that table was, "Gee, I wish there was some more."

Today the kids don't like *this*, they won't eat *that*, they can't stand the sight of the other ... with the result that they get a lopsided diet, because invariably they like the wrong things (like pop, candy, ice cream and potato chips) with the understandable undermining of their health.

Yes, no matter if the apologists for the processing and food chemical industries would have us believe we are the best fed people on earth and brimful of health, I think they're full of the stuff our farmers used to spread on their fields.

That is why I say ... no matter how you look at it, these kids today should be regarded with compassion, because they are the victims of conditions over which they have no control and had no part in creating — in an environment of a changing social structure and in a world that is on the brink of threatened disaster.

You may not go along with me, you may not like what I say, you may not like the way I say it, but can you honestly say it is not true?

## ARE YOU SANE OR NUTS?

I don't know who it was who said it, but it's always appropriate to attribute a saying to a wise and noble man ... so a wise and noble man once said, "The difference between insanity and genius is the thickness of a hair." Now you know why I don't mind being labelled "Nuts!"

Because I like my juices fresh — either directly from the orange or apple or freshly made with the juicer — my friends say I'm nuts! They buy their juices in cans and bottles and think their deplorable contents are the elixir of life.

When some little matter concerning my health goes askew, I sit and wonder why ... and I usually find out what my trouble is without any great difficulty. After all is said and done, what is simpler than putting your own house in order?

Therefore, as much as I respect some physicians, I seldom consult them. (My friends say I often insult them, but that isn't true!) And because I analyze my health problems myself, my friends say I'm nuts!

When my friends have a bellyache or a headache, instead of recognizing it as being caused by over-indulgence the night before, they run to their doctor. They're sane!

Because I believe that most of the processed foods we buy do not contain sufficient enzymes and minerals for a normal healthy person and therefore go to great lengths to get good variety and assortment in my foods, my friends say I'm nuts!

They go to a doctor and get a prescription and then go to a drug store and pick up their vitamins to bring or try to bring their bodies into balance. Of course, they're sane!

Because I eat nothing but fresh or dried raw fruit and grains every morning for breakfast . . . of course my friends again say I'm crazy!

They start off the day with cups of coffee, with cream and white sugar, and toast and vitamin-depleted cooked cereal . . . all without enough nutritional value to feed an ant . . . but of course they're sane.

Because I drink Red Clover Tea, Yerba Mate, Alfalfa Tea and other unprocessed herb drinks, some of my friends say I'm nuts!

They drink from five to ten cups of tea or coffee with or without milk, cream and white sugar, or half a dozen bottles of carbonated, chemically sweetened horrors . . . and they're sane.

Because I make sure I eat some raw food with every meal — either vegetable, fruit or grain, including plenty of raisins and dried prunes (and I'm as regular as a clock) — my friends say I'm nuts!

They take forced expulsion pills or milk of magnesia every night before retiring. They're sane!

Because I go to great lengths to get bread made out of pure whole wheat that isn't bleached, chemically treated or enriched, my friends say I'm nuts! They eat bread that's whiter than the freshly driven snow — chemically bleached

— with all the good taken out of it and various chemicals added to prevent it from ever going stale and to make it look pretty. They put that into their stomachs ... they're sane!

Because I snack with an apple or a slice of whole wheat or rye bread and unpasteurized honey, my friends say I'm nuts!

They have to have chocolate bars, a shot of liquor, a bottle of beer, a coke, a cigarette or a shot of some dope to pep them up.

They're sane!

## CRAZY BUT HEALTHY

This is a sort of crazy story, and I am not too sure that many of you will accept or believe it, but I was visiting a friend of mine and we were sitting and chatting about various things when eventually the topic got around to health ... as it invariably does. This friend was complaining that he had trouble with his shoulder. The doctor said he had bursitis. Then he had regular sieges of headaches and he mentioned, too, that his kidneys weren't functioning as well as they should.

I casually looked at him and said. "Well, if you ate the proper foods you wouldn't have any trouble."

His snort of derision and anger almost floored me. I didn't think a little fellow like this friend of mine could bellow so loudly ... "What the hell gives with you?" he rasped. "Don't you ever have any headaches and pains and aches?" And I said, "No, I don't — at least I haven't in years."

"That's utterly ridiculous," he snapped back. "I never heard of such a thing. Everybody gets sick and has aches and pains on and off."

"Now wait a minute," I said. "Do you mean that according to your concept of life and living a man must be sick and have pains and troubles and headaches?"

"Sure," he quipped, "as you get older you have all this trouble."

"Well, I can tell you that I don't, and I know many people my age and older who don't, and some who actually enjoy better health and vigor than I do . . . and I think I'm pretty peppy."

"I don't believe a word of it," he broke in; "it's not possible. A man is made to have pains and aches."

I didn't press the point any further. I realized I was up against a stone wall, so I let the matter drop.

It was quite a few weeks later when I dropped into the business place of this same friend. Evidently he had been thinking and the first thing he greeted me with was, "Tell me, what do you eat?" I sensed his interest and desire to be informed, so I outlined for his benefit my usual food pattern from morn till night. And here, for the benefit of all, I want to stress that I am not a vegetarian although I heartily endorse the vegetarian way of life and believe that it is the proper and right way. I also endorse the eating of as much uncooked food as possible because I have learned that only through the medium of uncooked foods, natural foods, do true health and well-being lie.

After I got through enumerating many of the natural foods that I eat, he said, "Bring me some of these on your next trip to the city."

"O.K.," I agreed. "Will I give you some advice and directions on their use?"

"Oh," he said, "you can give them to me when you bring the stuff."

"But," I said, "maybe I'd better tell your wife how to prepare them."

"Oh no," he put in. "I'm not taking them home; I'm going to eat these at work. If I took them home, my wife would laugh at me and tell me I was crazy."

So there you have it, folks . . . and I have found a similar pattern about foods wherever I talk to men. They are afraid their wives won't go for it . . . it would be too much trouble . . . it would cause them to be scoffed at and ridiculed, and that is one thing that most men cannot tolerate.

For those of you who are shut-ins or who know shut-ins or who have shut-ins as relatives and loved ones, may I offer a suggestion that may be of some material value?

If you can, get these shut-ins outside in a wheelchair or by some other means, so they can get some contact with the good earth. Either sit them with their feet in the earth or have them lie down on the earth. No, I don't mean on a blanket or on a bed or on a mattress. I mean to lie down on the grass or to sit on the grass. Better still have their bare feet contact the earth.

I think that the earth possesses tremendous beneficial and remedial qualities and they should be given a chance to manifest themselves ... especially to those who have been ailing for a long time.

If they cannot be brought outdoors, then by all means bring the good earth to them indoors in flats or in trays and have the shut-ins achieve the pleasure of planting a few seeds, and wherever possible have them do the potting themselves. Get them to have some positive contact with the good earth but please, no chemical fertilizers. Just plain ordinary wholesome soil from the bush or the meadow ... untainted by chemicals.

There is health in the good earth!

## AGRICULTURE, SOIL AND HEALTH

There is a positive link between the health of soil, the health of plants, the health of animals and the health of people.

A soil that is unbalanced or deficient can only grow plants that are unbalanced or deficient. It follows that such plants, if used for animal or human food, will create sick, ailing animals and humans. And if these animals are used as human food, they will in turn produce sick and ailing people. That's an immutable law that works every time. I have seen it clearly illustrated during my thirty years as a nurseryman.

It is further demonstrated clearly and unmistakably at Haughley in England. Here I make reference and give details from the annual report of The Haughley Experiment, 1963, New Bells Farm, Haughley, Stowmarket, Suffolk, England.

During a time when billions of dollars are being widely spent promoting the broad use of costly harmful chemical fertilizers, how does the common ordinary good earth fare? Listen to the Haughley story . . .

Twenty-five years ago a group of private people, who felt they might be paying too much attention to chemistry in our farming and too little to biology, began research on a farm scale in Suffolk to try to find out what effect, if any, different methods of management had upon the soil. They thought it might provide useful information on the relationship between the quality of food and ways of growing it. They felt that if such a relationship existed, it would probably be reflected in terms of health.

They divided the farm into three sections. On one, called 'the organic section', no fertilizers or sprays are used. It depends for its fertility upon farmyard manure, rough-composted with green weeds, and pasture mixtures including deep-rooting weeds. A second section, the 'mixed', was farmed in the conventional way, with farmyard manure, conventional pastures, and chemical fertilizers and sprays applied according to local practice. The third section is 'stockless', farmed without livestock, but with liberal applications of fertilizers and all organic matter derived from straw, stubble, etc., ploughed back.

Thus was born the Haughley Experiment, only such experiment on a field scale in the whole world. It did not set out to prove anything; only to try to learn what happens when you do or don't do certain things. It has now issued its first report.

It must be emphasized that this experiment can refer to only one farm in one part of England, so too much generalization would be rash. But the results are amazing.

Though it may sound strange to some the section to which no artificials have been applied shows no loss of fertility; in fact, fields at Haughley which have received no chemical manures for upwards of thirty years seem to be gaining in fertility, and this is reflected in the yields. On the other hand, yields in general on the organic section have been slightly less than on the mixed, and the pastures appear less luxuriant.

You will find at Haughley a small herd of Guernseys on each of these two sections, as nearly as possible identical, served by a common bull and managed in the same way. Each lives on the produce of its own section. One of the most consistent results has been that the 'organic' cows have yielded better than the 'mixed' cows and their total solids are slightly higher (12.5 per cent compared with 12.1 per cent). Moreover, the 'organic' herd has the better breeding record and eats less bulk of food. It looks as if the lower yields of the organic section could be more nourishing than the greater bulk of the other. Extended experiments on these lines are now contemplated.

The vital data and experience arising from Haughley after more than twenty-five years of continuous observation are invaluable, providing material that is available nowhere else.

You can obtain copies of this report for $1.00 U.S. or Canadian, from The Soil Association, 8F Hyde Park Mansions, Marylebone Road, London, N.W.1, England.

Here I would like to sound a sombre warning of things to come. I do not pretend to be a prophet but what I have seen with my own eyes convinces me that within a quarter of a century, but more likely within a decade, we in America will face starvation, famine and pestilence. The reason? Sustained chemical fertilization, spraying and dusting of our crops and their effect on our plant life is creating an imbalance in nature which in turn is effecting an ecological disruption in our insects, bacteria and fungi.

I have seen the signs in various crops — for example, in pineapples, avocados, sugar beets — where concentrated, continuous fertilization has been the rule. In most of these cases the outer appearance of the product is normal, but upon slicing it one finds that the core is rotted. The deterioration, in other words, is not apparent on the surface. The producer gets his money for the product but the consumer receives nothing of any value. And I say that this deep rooted imbalance in plants will grow by leaps and bounds.

To those of you who will say that you can prove that chemical fertilizers do give greater crop yields, I say, "Yes, but it is a short sighted view for they will give an increase in crops this year or the year following by robbing the soil of nutrients that nature intended to be given out over a period of ten, fifteen or twenty years".

Again, for proof of this assertion I would refer you to the Haughley experiment which has been in active existence for more than twenty five years. It gives clear adamant proof that in the long run the natural means is superior in every way to the chemical method.

You may ask why I say that the situation will all come to a head within twenty-five years. So, I will answer in this way. The use of chemical fertilizers began with Justus von Liebig back more than 100 years ago. He advocated and recommended the use of potassium-containing fertilizers and proved their value in the chemical laboratory and sold not millions, but billions of tons of chemical fertilizers. In fact, the billions of dollars that his potassium fertilizers brought into Germany helped the Kaiser wage World War I.

But listen to this — this is an eye-opener! When this same Justus von Liebig was given a plot of land by the elders of the Town of Giessen, he immediately put into practice the theories that he had advocated and that had sold billions of tons of potassium fertilizers. But strange to relate, while his promises and analysis and formulas worked to perfection in the test tube, when he sought to do the same on the land, they failed and failed miserably. He admitted his failure and I quote it here for you to read:

"I had sinned against the wisdom of the Creator, and received my righteous punishment. I wished to improve His work, and in my blindness believed that, in the marvellous chain of laws binding life on the earth's surface and keeping it always new, a link had been

63

forgotten which I, weak and powerless worm, must supply."
(From *Encyclopedia Britannica*,
Vol. XIV, P. 567, 1899 Edition)

He was therefore admitting that the chemical fertilization of soils was a positive failure. That is the reason that no fertilizers have been named after Liebig. In fact, the chemical people would prefer to forget all about him and they never refer to him because he recanted and admitted that what he sought to do was impossible.

Chemical fertilization has been practised for more than 100 years, but at a comparatively slow pace. It is only in the past quarter century that it has reached tremendous, gigantic, stupendous proportions. The sale of chemical fertilizers amounts to billions of tons and billions of dollars annually and it is so far-reaching that about 90 per cent of all crops on the North American continent, at least, are grown with and by means of chemical fertilizers and chemical sprays.

It is because of this great concentration, because of this tremendous spread of the use of chemical fertilizers and the effects that they have produced on our soils and crops and on our people that I base this prediction . . . within twenty five years, starvation, pestilence and disease will run havoc and be epidemic throughout America.

Now it may be your turn to ask me why I believe in the natural way of doing things — both in organic farming and gardening and in natural foods for my body. Why, you ask? Well, please listen and let me explain.

Because of my ignorance in former years, I paid out my hard-earned money to try the chemical way of farming. Yes, I even tried it too long. I was convinced by their propaganda and the efforts of the experimental stations that it was the right and proper thing to do . . . and only after some years of using chemical fertilizers, insecticides and sprays did I reach the positive conclusion that the natural way is the one and the right way.

I recall about fifteen years ago, one specific plot of

ground that I seeded to Chinese Elm. It so happened that this one year I was one of the few nurserymen throughout the country who had managed to get hold of some Chinese Elm seed and therefore, I wanted my seedlings to grow as large and vigorous as possible ... to harvest a crop of husky, lusty seedlings and get a better price for them.

I went to the experimental station and they recommended the fertilizer and the dosages. I followed them to the letter and I did get big, tall, leggy seedlings that were very succulent ... and as these were sold by size, I did very well. But the next year when I sowed a crop in that self-same plot, it was a failure. The following year the crop again was a failure — and the year after that, too. Practically nothing would produce a decent crop on that piece of soil until I brought in six big truck loads of soil from a farm that had been sold for industrial purposes. It was only after the soil was added that this plot of ground was brought back to normal.

I have fields on which I used weed killers, both the pre-emergent type and the regular. Crops were poor or failures on these lands as well ... until I allowed them to lie fallow for a few years and then sowed them to cover crop. I am not talking through my hat! I am talking from thirty years' experience.

Seeing my enthusiasm, you may ask, "If this natural method is so wonderful, why is it not better known throughout America?"

The answer is a simple one. The proponents of the natural methods do not have unlimited millions at their disposal to pay for advertisements in all the leading publications in the world, or for radio and television programs ... nor does their way of life permit such fabulous earnings.

It is not my intent to deny that chemistry has its place in this great universe of ours. Yes, it has its place in many niches and many segments of our society — but it does not have its place in our good earth or in our food and drink or in medicine. Furthermore, it is not my intent to stand before you and try to make you believe that every man who is a naturalist or who believes in the natural way of living or farming is a bright, upstanding, intelligent individual and the man who does chemical farming is the opposite . . . because again, that would not be true.

As I pointed out earlier in this chapter, chemicals can and do increase crop yields, but that is because the chemical fertilizers force into use and burn up and waste elements in the soil that will be required for crops five or ten or twenty years hence . . . but the chemical fertilizer people in their propaganda never ever dare mention this vital fact. But here and now let it be emphasized that chemical fertilizers at the start do produce increased yields and even amazing results on most farm projects. I am the first to admit this clear-cut result.

We also know of people today who were given drugs when they were ill and depressed due to a degeneration in their physical and mental condition. It helped sustain them over a difficult period. Now I have seen these drugs produce apparently sensational results, making the person bold and strong physically and mentally for a while . . . and some of them have become permanently addicted to drugs in this manner. But eventually, as everyone knows, the breakdown does occur and it is invariably deadly . . . and seldom do the addicted ever come out of it in good health.

So there we are. Would you advocate the use of drugs to people who are depressed or who have a headache or who are worried? Would you suggest the use of drugs for actors to help them give a better performance? Would you permit the use of drugs on race horses or other animals in order to get a greater effort from them? No, of course you wouldn't! Then why would you willingly and knowingly thus afflict the good earth?

Sure, you can get a greater burst of growth out of your soil by using chemical fertilizers . . . but the same yardstick applies to sick people, to horses, to actors and to the soil. You get a tremendous, energetic reaction by using these things but the end result is chaos and the wrecking of the physical properties of the soil, plant, beast and man.

# CHAPTER 5

## Proper Food

> *"Use your will power and better judgment to select and eat only the foods which are best for you, regardless of the ridicule or gibes of your friends or acquaintances."*
>
> .... DR. RICHARD T. FIELD

### TRIBUTE AND REFERENCE

In my search for the answers to the problems concerning human health and the proper diet of man, I have searched as diligently as my intelligence, my abilities and my eyes would permit. I have gone back in the literature of mankind to the beginning of the printed or written word and I am sincerely sorry to say that mankind's knowledge of the proper food for his health and well-being is woefully wanting. In fact, comprehension and information concerning proper food is most conspicuous because of its absence.

To me it is clear that the most worthwhile knowledge in the field of nutrition has only come to light in the past thirty years. Furthermore, I am sorry to say that even this knowledge is hidden, denied, lied about, exaggerated and corrupted ... so that only the most diligent student and investigator can find and learn the truth.

It is admitted that the Bible does give guidance concerning the proper food for man. In Genesis it tells us that the proper food for man is that food which Adam partook of in the Garden of Eden prior to the flood and by means of which man reached the age of almost 1,000 years. After the flood when man took to cooking his food, his life span dropped to 120 years. Later when he learned to use meat, his life span became the three score and ten which we know today.

However, throughout time there have been among us, men and women who sensed man's need for guidance. Greatest among these, in my humble opinion, was Ellen G. White. In her book, "The Ministry of Healing," there is a chapter on diets and health. In this chapter is given some of the finest nutritional advice ever written by anyone. Just think ... this gifted, inspired lady possessed this tremendous knowledge, more than sixty five years ago!

Even in the light of our present supposedly great scientific achievements and knowledge, most of the scientists and nutritionists are floundering about. Yet without the vital, newly-gained scientific knowledge, this woman laid down the soundest principles of health and nutrition ever written by anybody. My study of her writing on food and nutrition leads me to believe that this woman was a beacon of light in a troubled, strained, floundering world. If only more people would read and follow her teachings, the world would be a much better place in which to live.

Admittedly, I find one or two small principles on which I differ or disagree with her ... but then, I have before me scientific knowledge gained since that time and which was not available to her. May I suggest to my readers who are not acquainted with the writings of this great religious and health leader that they read "The Ministry of Healing," or at least the chapter on diets and health.

Let me further emphasize that this advice is not based on any desire on my part to lead you into any religious beliefs or teachings. In this book I deal strictly with food and health. I prefer to leave religion to the clergy. However, I feel that I would be remiss in my duties as an author if I did not call your attention to a memorable piece of work in the field of nutrition ... a work that, in my opinion, ranks among the best.

## WHAT TO EAT

Knowing what to eat, in my opinion, is probably the most difficult task that faces a human being.

It is as easy as pie to follow your father or your grandfather in their eating habits. In fact, that's just about what 90% or more of the people throughout the world do. And if you are an observer of any discernment, you will quickly reflect that this hasn't been a very successful or wise pattern to follow.

Yes, I recognize that many of us had parents who lived to the three score and ten, and beyond, in comparative good health ... but believe me, they were the exception rather than the rule.

For example, take my own father. He lived to be seventy ... but was killed by a motor car while crossing the street. The autopsy performed after his death revealed that his arteries, his heart and his body and organs in general were in good physical condition. So you would assume that if I followed my father's eating habits I'd be comparatively safe and would lead a good, healthy life and live to be seventy or more. True ... but I also reflect that my father suffered very many aches and pains — from his back, from his feet and other things. I don't think I'd want to follow that pattern and lead a life that had so many pains and aches, even if it did permit me to live out my allotted span.

But the overflowing graveyards with markers indicating that most died long before seventy are testimony to the fact that many of our parents were not quite as fortunate. Therefore, I would suggest that you do not look to your parents or your predecessors for a guide as to what to eat. Take time to inform yourself through readily available literature as to the proper food and way of life for health and longevity.

Here I must make a most serious and alarming statement, based on my observations and studies of facts and statistics. Most children — boys, girls and even many young men and women of today — will never reach 70 or even 60 or 50. Why? Because of the heavy loads of chemicals in their bodies accumulated from the chemically treated food and drink they consume, plus the harmful effects of smoking and other contaminants. These chemicals will cause various forms of cancer and many other killing diseases.

Knowing how to live must take into account what to eat ... and on that score most people know little or nothing. Yes, it is a grim tragedy that when it comes to food and health they take the attitude, "Oh, let the doctor worry. That's what I pay him for."

When I see a man take that attitude (and there are many) then I know for certain that man will die before his time — or lead a life of illness and debility. The most important single factor that governs a human being's health is knowing what to eat and following that precept. Now I did not say that it is the only factor involved, but it is the most important one because without the proper food all other principles, practices and philosophies concerning health will come to naught.

Now you may ask, "What is the proper food to eat?" . . . and I want to tell you, friends, that is not an easy question to answer.

Broadly speaking, there are two widely accepted schools of thought on eating. One is the omnivorous way of life. In this case the diet would include meats, fruits, vegetables, grains, nuts and anything that can be procured or is deemed fit to eat. The second and I submit. the more difficult way of life is the vegetarian.

I find it convenient when referring to vegetarians and their way of life to divide them into three distinct groups, as follows:

A. The strict vegetarians who use no animal products whatsoever. This excludes eggs and dairy products, but includes cooked vegetable products, bread and other baked goods.

B. The lacto-ovo vegetarians who use milk or other dairy products, as well as eggs, along with the foods in the vegetable kingdom.

C. Then there is a lesser known and still lesser understood philosophy on eating — commonly known as the "raw fooders" in my lexicography. Those who follow this way of life partake of no animal food (flesh) but do utilize the so-called "fruit" of the animal . . . that is, dairy or milk products such as milk, cheese and eggs. And as the name indicates, they eat no cooked, baked, treated or fired food whatsoever.

But there is also an offshoot of the above — the "ultra raw fooder" who eats no animal food of any kind. He is really making life hard for himself . . . but perhaps beautiful.

Now I want to clarify my position. I am not a vegetarian, although I have for more than a quarter of a century recognized the truism that vegetarianism is the sanest and most elevated way of life, the cleanest way of life and most certainly the most moral way of life. But I also recognize that being a strict vegetarian . . . that is, eating no animal products whatsoever . . . is difficult, especially for those of us who live in the temperate zone. It is much easier to be a true vegetarian and live in California or some other tropical or semi-tropical part of the world. If one were to dwell there I am sure one would find no problem being a vegetarian. But here, where I live, where I would say we have five months of winter a year, then I take sanctuary with animal foods.

I have no doubt that the vegetarian way of life was the way of life ordained by nature. But then, perhaps a benign nature intended that human beings live in the tropics or semi-tropics.

I believe that for proper living in the northern latitudes the use of meat, fowl or fish is fully justifiable and one meal every day should have a normal portion of meat, fowl or fish, preferably broiled and never fried. The alternative is to become a raw fooder . . . but this way of life is both difficult and unacceptable to most. The reason I place great emphasis upon "meat" or "raw food" is that the vegetarian way of eating cooked and heat treated vegetables can only lead to debility, disease and a shortened life span.

A warning! If you do eat meat and fowl, seek to obtain meat and fowl that has not been treated with diethylstilbestrol. This may be very hard to do but if the meat you eat has been so treated (and most of it is) then you are impairing your health. You would be far better off if you eliminated all meat from your diet at once.

Here is the way I would rank the health and long life of the four classes mentioned above. First and foremost, the raw fooders. The omnivorous type is next. They live as long, or almost as long, as the raw fooders but they suffer more chronic and other illnesses. As third I would rank the vegetarians who do not follow the raw food system and in fourth place I would put the lacto-ovo vegetarians.

One of the most vital aspects in diet, and this is especially important to the vegetarians, is that the diet be as varied as humanly possible. This, my friends, involves considerable effort and difficulty. From my travels in most countries of the world I would go on record as saying that it is virtually impossible to get a balanced diet as a vegetarian outside of America.

Even among those who follow the natural way of life there is widespread disagreement as to the right way to eat and the proper foods. Yes, this even occurs among the vegetarians, as you can readily understand, but it goes deeper than I have indicated above. For example, one group of vegetarians claims that the right food of the vegetable kingdom is fruit alone. Some condescend to say fruit and nuts but they will go no further . . . and all other forms of vegetable food are taboo. They even claim that the grains are harmful and that vegetables are meant for cows, horses and other beasts . . . and they attempt to bring forth argument and evidence in various forms to prove their point.

I have devoted considerable time and study to their arguments and I cannot hold that the fruitarian way of life is the right way. My opinion is that anything in the plant kingdom that is suited or fit to eat is fair game and the broader the variety the better.

Then there is the school that advocates that certain foods should only be eaten with certain other foods. This branch of nutrition is quite a science in itself and is known as "food combining." For example, its exponents might maintain that melons should be eaten alone or that you should not mix carbohydrates with proteins or fats with carbohydrates. These discourses and arguments appear to go on endlessly.

Then there is the school that maintains that the mono diet is the only correct form of eating. With this line of thinking I fall in line, for my studies reveal that by eating one food only at a specified meal you get optimum results and your digestive system would never be taxed and thus remain in top condition. Who can deny that the mono diet is the sanest and most sensible way of eating and would be most beneficial to the human system? But on the other hand, who, who has lived to be forty or fifty years of age and tasted various foods in combination, could ever tolerate or exist on a mono diet? The thought of eating only bananas for one meal, rice for another meal, potatoes for the next, and so on would make me want to end it all there and then.

I have always been and still am a gourmet. I love good food and I love dining in the company of pleasant people. But what fancy dining can a man do on raw vegetables, fruits, grains and nuts? Not much, you say, and I must agree. But mind you, I still am invited out and I visit many people who prepare some very attractive delectable meals of raw fruits and vegetables . . . but they also usually have some cooked foods for those who prefer them or because the cook likes them.

Every time I mention the optimum health diet of completely raw foods without fragmentation to my friends, they immediately say, "Oh, well, that's a cinch . . . no cooking, no trouble, just eat!"

Well, that isn't true. My experience has shown me that it is more trouble to prepare these unfired dishes than it is the conventional cooked dishes. You can prepare a very nice tasty meal by putting a steak on the grill and fixing a few mashed potatoes. There you've got a full-fledged meal according to American standards . . . that is, assuming you've got butter and white bread all set and some frozen peas and some canned fruit and baked goods. It doesn't take much time or preparation to set up a table with dead, nutritionless food like that on it.

Yes, the way of the transgressor is hard. I presume that I am the transgressor because when you eat the way you should eat for health and long life, the road is indeed rough . . . for you are battling against accepted and widely practised standards. It may be all right for those who have become accustomed to it or began it when they were young, but I've only taken to it wholeheartedly in the past few years. And I do admit that the going is grim. But the amount of energy and pep that I have, the fact that I feel in the pink of condition and display it, makes the task and the effort worthwhile.

So there you have it! I've laid before you a little bit about what to eat. I'm leaving the choice in your hands. However, I must pass on to you my recommendations and I am going to tell you exactly what I eat. I am sixty-five years of age and a check-up by a top ranking naturopath, herbalist, chiropractor, osteopath dropped the verdict that I am in perfect health and have the heart of a lion.

I don't want this to sound as though I were bragging, but I have boundless energy. I don't know what it means to be tired. I am physically and mentally capable of doing more work than when I was thirty years of age and I'll stand up to any man my age and even younger. It is my positive conviction that a proper diet is the answer.

Finding a satisfying as well as healthful diet was not a light task. I have long known that the vegetarian way of life was right and proper by all aesthetic standards, but how to accomplish this task was the problem. I have known, watched and studied vegetarians and vegetarianism for some years and do not regard vegetarians as a robust or healthy group. However, my studies of health and nutrition revealed the fact that a diet of raw grains, fruits and vegetables was the optimum for health and long life. Therefore, I resolved that until I was sure that my knowledge about food was adequate, I would move cautiously.

I won't try to tell you to follow my diet or my way of

living but for those of you who want to know what my diet is, here it is . . .

*Breakfast*

A raw apple or other area fruit in season and two to four heaping tablespoonfuls of my special breakfast concoction.

Without boasting or exaggerating, it is the finest, the best balanced, the most nutritious assembled food in the whole world.

| | |
|---|---|
| Rolled whole oats | 10 parts |
| Rolled whole barley | 2 parts |
| Rolled whole wheat | 2 parts |
| Rye | 2 parts |
| Buckwheat | 2 parts |
| Millet | 2 parts |
| Sesame | 1 part |
| Flax | 1 part |
| Alfalfa herb, powdered | 2 parts |
| Dried Prunes | 2 parts |
| Dried Raisins | 2 parts |
| Dried Peaches | 1 part |
| Dried Apricots | 2 parts |
| Dried Dates | 1 part |
| Dried Figs | 1 part |
| Total — 15 ingredients | |

Cut fruits into small pieces. Thoroughly mix fruits and grains together.

Don't cook or heat . . . just add water — spring or well water preferred . . . let soak overnight.

Add milk, cold or warm (never hot), if desired. Eat two to five tablespoonfuls every day or at least every other day.

I make a batch to last about a week. Keep it in the refrigerator.

After you have felt and recognized its benefits, switch to whole, unbroken grains (oats, barley, wheat) for optimum results.

Maybe fifteen ingredients are not essential at one time.

But remember, I am trying to help busy people keep healthy by means of proper, natural, uncooked, untreated food in this modern day.

Make certain that none of these grains or fruits have been treated, steamed, sulphured or otherwise chemically violated.

*Lunch*

Salad, composed of these vegetables — all raw — many or all, as available (I like variety) — and preferably broken, not cut . . .

| | | |
|---|---|---|
| Celery | Lettuce | Cucumber |
| Endive | Tomato | Green Pepper |
| Onion | Kohlrabi | Mushroom |
| Carrot | Cabbage | Artichoke |
| Garlic | Celeriac | Cauliflower |
| Fennel | Parsley | Zucchini Squash |
| Radish | Spinach | Green Peas |
| Beets | Broccoli | Dandelion Greens |
| Dill | Avocado | Sweet Red Pepper |
| Corn | Parsnip | Asparagus |
| Cress | Turnip | Swiss Chard |
| Okra | Eggplant | Mustard Greens |

Sprinkle with raisins, flax, sesame and sunflower seeds. Add honey or blackstrap molasses in place of dressing. No other dressing or salt or pepper.

The flax and other seeds take the place of oil. Use cold pressed vegetable oil, if you must, and unpasteurized cider vinegar.

For between-meal snacks — any fruit in season or dried fruit, dates, figs, raisins, prunes, apricots, peaches or nuts.

*Dinner*

Raw salad
Meat or fish (roasted, stewed or broiled)
Homemade soup (occasionally)

*Before-Retiring Snack*
  Banana or other fresh fruit

*Important Notes*
  No cooking of any fruit. Prunes or other dried fruits are delectable steeped in water, alone or in mixture.
  If you enjoy or need cooked vegetables like potatoes, squash and others, use them only for the evening meal.
  All vegetables should be organically grown and unsprayed if possible, but I admit this is difficult.
  No pork.
  Meat broiled, stewed, roasted, but not fried.
  Dairy products keep to a minimum, and wherever possible unpasteurized. Cottage cheese is a fragmented food ... may be a good filler but a poor food nutrition-wise as most elements were lost in the whey.
  Eat seeds, nuts, grains whole wherever possible.
  Fruits, vegetables, grains, seeds and nuts are your best foods without exception. Make them the major or the most important part of your diet.
  Avoid salt and processed condiments.
  Bread should be made only from whole grain untreated flour.
  Never use white sugar. Honey is the best sweetening agent, next is raw sugar, then maple sugar and molasses.
  One can still live naturally and enjoy all of the essentials for health and long life. Adequate supplies of good natural foods are available twelve months a year. Properly stored root crops like potatoes, carrots, parsnips, onions, turnips, beets, artichokes, kohlrabi, celeriac and many others are found on the shelves of most food shops throughout the country. One can find most fresh green items imported from California, Texas, Florida and other places that contain adequate quantities of wholesome, natural, nutritional food values; for example, lettuce, celery, cabbage, cauliflower, cucumbers, broccoli, brussels sprouts, endive, peppers, spinach, tomatoes, green peas. Then, too, fruits and nuts like pears, apples, oranges, grapefruit, lemons, walnuts, pignolias, brazils, butternuts,

77

filberts, pecans, almonds, hickory nuts and peanuts are generally available. Then there are the grains that are indigenous to the north — barley, rye, wheat, oats, buckwheat and millet — all of which make good healthful eating.

Among all fruits in America, nuts are the most generally organically grown (a) because they are deep tap rooted and draw their nourishment from way down in the subsoil and (b) because spraying is not usually called for or plausible.

If you prefer meat and fish, there is a wide variety available twelve months a year. Most of the packaged meats and fish of course have been processed and thus treated with a wide variety of chemicals for various purposes. Concerning meat (be it fresh, cooked, smoked or processed) in most cases an injurious chemical has been surreptitiously placed in the feed of the animal. The same applies to chicken and turkey. They contain a most harmful chemical, diethylstilbestrol, which is not eliminated by cooking. If you were following the natural way of life, you would either have to give up meat and poultry or find a source of supply procured from untreated animals.

Home canning and preserving used to be a vital part of the way of life in bygone years but because the canning process involves cooking and the destruction of the enzymes, this method is frowned upon by most of the knowledgeable nutritionists who follow the natural way of living.

Frozen foods, if completely without chemical treatment, are much better nutritionally than canned foods ... but not nearly as good as fresh foods.

It must be remembered that no food was ever improved by cooking and it is no exaggeration to state categorically that uncooked and untreated food is the best. One may like cooked foods, one may prefer them, but that does not mean that they are of any great nutritional value to the body. The fact is that uncooked foods, foods in the natural state without cooking or chemical treatments contain much higher nutritional values than cooked foods.

During my quest for knowledge in the field of nutrition and health, I have read through hundreds of volumes, thousands of articles, brochures, pamphlets and booklets. I have studied many volumes of chemistry, biochemistry and other scientific and academic works on nutrition and food and food processing.

From this monumental rubble of pseudo-knowledge I have not found a bit of proof that the nutrient value of any cooked or processed food has ever been positively established. I repeat ... even at the risk of boring you, because I deem this of great importance ... that nowhere is there any conclusive laboratory proof that cooked or processed foods are of significant nutritional value to the body.

Please bear in mind that I am familiar with the fact that man has lived in a form of pseudo-health for thousands of years on a diet consisting chiefly of cooked foods. I contend that the fact that he does live to anything resembling true old age is definitely credited to the small amount of raw food that composed part of his food intake in that period ... which in most cases consisted of fruits like apples or citrus and perhaps a bit of dried fruit and some vegetables. Therefore, it is that little bit of unfired food that he puts into his system that actually sustains him.

Raw foods will be accepted, digested and assimilated by the body of any normal, healthy person without any apparent great effort by the body itself. This is achieved by a system that nature has evolved during the time that human beings have occupied the earth. In simple parlance, nature knows how to handle, assimilate and distribute raw food to the body. When the human body is restricted to an entirely cooked food diet, which is the case with many people due to impairment of digestion or some other condition, it is tantamount to slow death. This is my warning to those who try to live on a mainly cooked food diet.

I do not suggest that the human body is incapable of getting anything of value from cooked foods. I just want to go on record as claiming that the amount of nutrients that the body can derive from cooked food is minimal and if that were all that the body received, it would soon end in disaster.

I place cooked foods, processed foods, devitalized foods, chemically treated foods, preserved and enriched foods all in the same category ... as foods unfit for human consumption. They may look or taste good to our perverted appetites but any man who will take the trouble to investigate will quickly learn that these corrupted, degraded foods can only lead to degeneration, debility and an early grave.

It must be forcibly stressed that a diet consisting wholly of raw fruits and vegetables cannot long sustain the human body in good health because both fruits and vegetables contain insufficient quantities of essential oils. Let me stress, raw fruits and vegetables do contain some oils but, in my opinion, not enough.

Most people make use of various oils such as corn, sunflower, linseed, cottonseed, safflower, olive and other oils. The best I can say for these oils or fats, even if they be cold-pressed, is that they are perhaps better than no oil at all. However, and I stress this, the way to get our oils is by means of grains, seeds and nuts ... all of which are amply provided with these vital, essential, natural fats. These vital oils are at your disposal when you eat these grains, seeds and nuts without fragmenting or destroying them.

Therefore, along with your diet of adequate quantities of fruits and vegetables, be sure to include an ounce or two of grains, seeds or nuts every single day. In this way you will get the proper fats in perfect, natural form so they can be completely digested and assimilated by your body.

It is my belief that fats or oils are essential. The human body cannot long exist in good health without them. But get them just as nature intended and provided them.

## HEAR YE, HEAR YE ...

Listen, ye non-believers, ye of little faith, ye of stubborn mind, ye of failing bodies, ye who are steeped in ignorance ... listen and learn.

I tell you that a cooked-food-fed body is a diseased body and conversely, a raw-food-fed body is a healthy body. And knowledge cannot help but lead you to health and long life.

I will illustrate my points succinctly if you wish proof. Take two fresh eggs. Boil one of them. Then crack open the fresh egg that has not been boiled and crack open the egg that has been boiled. Put your nose close to them and smell them. The fresh, uncooked egg will smell wholesome and even fragrant, but the cooked egg will have a noticeable unpleasant, varying sulphury odor ... in truth, it stinks!

This is but a simple bit of proof to indicate to you that cooking makes undesirable chemical changes in all of the foods that you eat.

You cannot long remain healthy on a diet that consists chiefly or primarily of cooked foods. You must include a fair to large portion of uncooked fruits, grains, vegetables and nuts in your diet if you will avoid the onslaught of degenerative diseases and untimely death.

Arthritis is labelled as a disease that can affect and afflict only those who eat chiefly cooked foods. No person or animal that eats only or chiefly raw foods can have arthritis.

## LET THE EARTH BRING FORTH GRASS

Even among the vegetarians and hygienists or the naturopaths there appears to be no agreed upon ways and means of life ... that is, in regard to food.

One school of thought says that the proper food for man is fruit, another says fruit and vegetables. A third group claims that all that nature provides is for man — fruits, nuts, grains and even the fungi.

Now it is immaterial which school of thought you belong to and there is argument pro and con as each of these groups can produce testimony to bear out, or as they maintain, prove their beliefs.

From my studies and searchings it appears that the

native and other grasses have never played a part in the life of man for food and I have wondered about this but could reach no conclusion as to why this form of natural food was omitted.

From a casual glance I would say because animals like the cow, deer, goat, sheep and all the so-called grazing creatures partook of grass or found grass the ideal food for them, man assumed that what was good for a cow wasn't good enough for him and therefore left the grammaceous plants alone. The more I observe, the more I study, the greater becomes my conviction that the grasses are good food, probably as good as most or maybe even among the best — although I would not expect you to choose a blade of nicely mown lawn grass over and above a peach, an apple, a pear, a mango, a papaya or a banana. But, nutritionally, I'd be willing to bet real money that the grasses contain as much food value per ounce, in fact much more than any of the best fruits that you can mention.

I do realize that we have been consuming leafy vegetables and the nutritionists recommend them very highly for their high food value, but the grasses are from an entirely different family and they have been excluded, avoided or ignored. So I am suggesting to all of you who will listen, "Give thought to grass as food for man. It may be the answer to your health problem."

It is abundant. It is self-sowing. It is self-maintained. It is rich in all the nutrients required to sustain the human body. Therefore, it is a good natural food.

It requires no preparation. It is available twelve months of the year. It never loses its food value. It doesn't have to be treated and will not spoil in any way. It is available in wide variety — in color, texture, flavor and nutrient value.

Yes, too, I have heard scientists claim that grass is no good for a human being because we do not possess the stomach of a ruminant or the gastro-intestinal bacteria required to properly digest, break down or assimilate these grasses. It is claimed by them that the cows or even birds have a different kind of digestive system. I suggest that this is just humbug and nonsense. If we eat grass and gradually break into it by taking small quantities, by degrees, the gastro-intestinal bacterial flora will be developed as required for proper digestion and assimilation. For example, a pig eats grass, grain, vegetables, fruits, nuts, tubers — yes, and meat too — and if you know man you will realize that he is a bigger hog than a pig... he eats everything, too!

## SHODDY OR TODDY

Drink your way to health! This is addressed to those of you who are seeking to recover or regain health that has somehow managed to slip away through the years.

How many of us are there who just mosey about in this circus of life — not paying any particular attention to any set rules or laws of health and well-being? We go about eating what we like, sleeping when we like, doing what we like... and if somewhere in our wanderings, we falter and find that we're not as strong or as virile or as healthy as we would be... we just assume that it's age; that it's time taking its toll.

Listen to me friends... time does take its toll, but time has enduring patience. It has all the time in the world. It's not rushing you or crowding you, or telling you to hurry up because the grim reaper is waiting. There is no need to hurry the grim reaper... for as I said above, time is something that he's loaded with.

Therefore, if you are not as peppy or as lively as you think you should be... talk to yourself, ask yourself a few sensible questions. The first question that I want you to ask yourself is this... "Is the food that I am putting into my system living food?" By living food, I mean food that is truly alive; that contains enzymes and living bacteria, and all other micro-organisms, just as nature intended. You see, nature meant for us all to eat only living food, and let me tell you... canned food, cooked food, processed food, colored food and such are all dead. There is not a spark of life in any of them.

So what can you expect from dead food other than

death? No one on earth has the power to turn the dead back into the living, so therefore, if you want health, use food that is alive, and you in turn will get life from it. Why should you be content to take your grape juice, your apple juice, carrot juice, pineapple juice, tomato juice from a can when you know that it is dead? It has been treated; it has been contaminated, it is boiled until no spark of living organism remains. So I'm going to ask again ... what can you expect from dead food?

The fact that the old school of nutritionists and most modern nutritionists do not tell you that is not my fault. I ask you to read, to study and to judge for yourself. No, there is nothing, absolutely nothing on earth that can take the place of living, natural, wholesome food.

The best way to get the full benefit that is contained in an apple is to eat an apple; but if you want the effects quickly and easily, the next best thing is to drink the juice ... but the *live* juice! The same applies to an orange, a grapefruit, tomatoes, pineapple and many or any other fruits and vegetables. The quickest way to get the best out of them, and to derive health and well-being from them is to drink the fresh juice. Therefore, it is my belief from actual experience that one of the simplest and most commonsense ways on earth to derive the health that is contained within those marvelous fresh fruits and vegetables is to drink the fresh juice.

But why pay high prices that these juices would cost you when by the use of a juicing machine or juice extractor, you can perform that simple miracle right in your own home ... at your convenience and with ease and comfort. A bushel of apples will give you gallons of delicious, fresh, health-giving, wholesome apple juice. A bushel of carrots will give you carrot juice by the gallon, and a bushel of tomatoes will give you enough juice to have a bath in ... all for a few cents. If you went into a shop and bought this juice ... the fresh would be almost impossible to get ... even the canned juice would cost you many, many times the price of the real, genuine, wholesome, fresh juice that you would get by means of your own juicer.

Get yourself a juicer ... make this test. Taste the canned apple juice or orange juice, and then drink your home-made juice from your own juicer ... you and you alone be the judge. You know what? You'll never drink anything but fresh juice again as long as you live. You'll wonder what in blazes that other stuff is anyway ... it will certainly have no resemblance to the fresh, wholesome juice that you will be getting from your own juicer ... and the health that will follow in its wake is yours to have and to hold for many added years!

Authorities say that one's system may be starving for the minerals, the enzymes and the vitamins contained in a table full of raw vegetables — especially those of you who have denied yourself these health-giving raw fruits and vegetables through the years. But who has the stomach capacity big enough to eat a table full of raw vegetables even if your system does crave and need them? But a juicer can render that table full of vegetables into such a form that by drinking a quart or two of juice a day, you will have most of the valuable vitamins, minerals and enzymes contained within them; and you will not have had to force that huge bulk upon yourself.

So it is by the simple expedient of reducing that wholesome tableful of fruits and vegetables to juice that you have solved the vital problem of giving the body the health-giving nutrients that it has been denied and that it needs. It is my sincere belief that fresh, wholesome fruit juice is one of the simplest and most direct roads to health known to either science or laymen.

Dr. Risser, noted Pasadena bone specialist, states, "Infantile paralysis can be prevented by a diet rich in Vitamin C." The following juices are rich in Vitamin C ... tomato, apple, orange, lemon, grapefruit and, of course, many other fruits and vegetables.

## MUMBO-JUMBO AND ABRACADABRA

There are a goodly number of my friends and relatives who through the years have had to consult their doctors because of heart attacks or other serious illnesses and they were hospitalized. Then when they were about to go home to convalesce, the doctors invariably tell them, "Don't worry about what you eat. Just make sure you get a balanced diet."

You see, friends have passed this information on to me for many years. In fact, many of my doctor friends have told me that that is what they usually advise their patients to do. And when I hear this I invariably grit my teeth and scowling like an umpire grimacing "You're out!" I say, "What the hell do you mean by a balanced diet?"

Well, they usually latch on to the prescribed conglomeration of phrases about proteins, carbohydrates and fats and vitamins and minerals and calories until I say to them, "Why in blazes don't you just say you don't know what you're talking about? You learned those phrases in your early days at medical school and you've never understood them, you've never had them explained to you and even the guy who taught them to you couldn't explain them. You wouldn't know what a balanced diet was if it was scrambled out before you on a palette or plate . . . and for that matter, neither would 999 people out of 1,000."

Now I'm not crying about man's ignorance or trying to belittle the medical profession because when it comes to ignorance, I've got more than my share. Yet it is high time that someone did explain to someone else exactly what is meant by a balanced diet. And I'll be the first to lend a listening ear!

## FALSE FICKLE FRIENDLY FIRE GOD

I don't know how long it is since man first began the use of herbs. Hundreds of years — yes, thousands of years easily. I have herbals that date back to 1600 . . . and Dioscorides goes back to the first century A.D. . . . and Theophrastus four hundred-odd years before that.

But herbs were mentioned in Greek and Roman writings, as well as ancient Chinese and Sanskrit too — surely they go back 5,000 years anyway. The use of herbs easily antedates the written word or the spoken word for that matter. There isn't the faintest reason to doubt that they even reach into the time when man first found he needed something to help him with his health problems.

It is therefore apparent that herbs have been food and medicine for man for thousands of years — if not since man first looked to the fields and forests and orchards for his food.

In the natural way of things, I doubt if the Lord or nature intended medicine to be medicine and food to be food. In my simple mind food and medicine always were, always have been and always will be . . . one.

Obviously they were cleft apart or separated by someone or some group for their own reasons. The fact that man has remained on this earth and that his numbers grew and that he spread to all parts of the world is clearly indicative that man can live and heal himself by the herbs of the fields and the forests, as well as those from the streams and the seas.

Somehow, through the years I have been unable to understand man's abandonment of natural herbs as food and medicine. You see, to me it seems that nature and herbs and trees and health all fit together in a simple beautifully woven pattern. When I read and saw through the past century or more the abandonment and the desertion of man of his herbs, it seemed incongruous. Where had nature failed? I just couldn't understand it.

But the years bring light, discernment and understanding . . . and now I begin to see why man was so easy to lure away from the old reliables.

One of the most vital and valuable herbs, food or medicine that we have in creation is garlic. Say what you like — laugh at it — joke about it — but garlic still remains a most vital food and cure-all in most parts of the world. It's not used too much in the Western world . . . or should I say in America . . . because of our sensitive proboscis. We can stand the smell that emanates from the mouth of a hiccoughing alcoholic or the belchings of a beer-bellied guzzler. But the fair aroma of garlic emanating from the ruby lips of a fair damsel would turn your amorous instincts into a fizzling fiasco, to say the least. However, if both you and your sweetheart had a bit of garlic on your breath, you wouldn't notice it at all. In fact, your breath would be to each other ... kissing sweet!

It is also true that garlic has its best effect and does its best culinary work in salads ... in plain words, when used raw.

In reading the herbals — whether written by Gerrard back in 1600 or by Parkinson, Culpepper, Salmon *et al* in the 1700's and 1800's or by one of the ancients, Theophrastus, Dioscorides and others — one finds they always tell of plucking the herbs fresh and then using them in poultices, unguents, teas or brews ... but always, it seems, heated, stewed or boiled in water.

When man learned to fire his foods it was the beginning of his degradation; when he took up the boiling of his health-restoring healing herbs that was the *coup de grâce*.

From the information and research laid down by modern scientists, it would appear that some little known things called enzymes have entered the picture. No one seems to know very much about them or what they are or where they come from or why. But science is taking a second and a third look into these protein catalysts, micro-organisms or whatever else they might be termed.

One thing they do know about them is that wherever they are things begin to happen and never stop happening. But they have also learned that when you heat them to 120 degrees, you kill most of them . . . and at boiling-point hardly a sign of an enzyme is left!

Yet somehow, if you want to make sure that a job of nutrition is done or any other job where nature acts, there must be enzymes. Well, there isn't any great quantity of enzymes around when you brew, stew or concoct something with boiling water. On the other hand, when herbs are used externally, they are invariably used in their raw or natural state . . . and I expect that the results, when the herbs are used in this manner, are great or spectacular because they are filled with enzymes and the enzymes immediately go to work.

Perhaps the herbals need to be rewritten and the remedies in which herbs are used should call for them not to be boiled, but to be cut up or grated and used steeped or uncooked. That the herbs have the attributes claimed for them by the herbalists, I do not deny or even doubt. And if they were given a chance to perform their functions as nature intended — that is, uncooked — I suspect that the results obtained or the cures effected might be spectacular. Think it over.

I guess you've learned by now that I have some really balmy ideas — ideas that don't make sense at all to some people. And is it any wonder?

Yet I am not so deep or profound that my theories would be difficult for the average grade eight man or woman to understand. I have believed that when mankind first learned to use a fire and cook his food, he cut a goodly number of years from his life and impaired his strength, his vitality and his health.

Cooking, of course, is tantamount to ruining food or lessening its value or nutrient content ... apart from killing the enzymes that would make it readily available to body tissues.

Then, through the years that I have been reading and studying matters concerning health, food and medicine and herbs, I've reached the conclusion that the herbalists went off the beaten path or beam, I should say, when they stopped using their herbs in their natural, uncontaminated, unprepared state. As long as they used the herbs as they came from the field, they performed quite efficiently and effectively. But when they began to cook and stew and boil and concoct these herbs, then I suspect that the herbs lost some or most of their potency.

I have reached the conclusion that to benefit from these herbs to their fullest extent, they should wherever possible be used without cooking or boiling. I would steep the herb, if necessary, or powder it and water it down — mix it with something palatable, if it is itself unpalatable. But I would not boil or stew it. Steep it, I would, and use the juice ... or better still, the juice and the solids ... and, to my belief and understanding, you would be getting the full effective force of the natural values contained within the herb.

My reason is simple: "Boiling or extreme heat kills enzymes and needed bacteria and micro-organisms."

Most certainly I understand and believe that this is not the accepted technique and isn't done by any or most herbalists. Yet this is what I believe.

## NIPPY NORTH, SUNNY SOUTH

It is my solemn conviction that the food found in the north is for people who live in the north and food that is grown in the south is for people who live in the south.

You may, however, say that that is all right for animals because they have no means of getting south for their food during the winter but that man can go there. But that is my main point of argument. Nature provided for her offspring, be they insects, animals or humans, so they did not have to go south. In fact, nature assumed that it was not feasible. Therefore, everything required for the health and sustenance of life in the north is provided in the north.

Nature in her wisdom placed all of the required nourishment, complete and whole, in the food that was indigenous to that climate. You will find health and long life eating the natural products of your own area or the district in which you live.

Of course, this depends on whether or not you will return the wastes back to the land from which you claimed them.

## DEAD OR ALIVE

Life begets life, and death begets I don't know what.

I'm trying to say that if you want to be alive, healthy and well and full of energy, then it is essential that you guard your health, and above all — eat living food. How can dead food give you life and energy?

What do I mean by dead food? Well, let's check into the average morning meal.

Your beverage has been boiled or cooked, and it is as dead as a doornail. The white sugar that you use was dead before it ever came into your home. The cream or milk that you use in your coffee, if it isn't already dead, is dying because of the pasteurization process it was put through. The same applies to your butter or margarine which is even worse.

So you have some toast made out of dead bread, and of course, the toasting process only helps to cremate it. Then you might have some jam or jelly (boiled and sterilized so that not a spark of life remains). Who knows — you may even have a breakfast of eggs and bacon cooked to a frazzle so that not one living enzyme or micro-organism remains alive.

But perhaps you're different! You may have had some cereal — maybe oatmeal, wheaties or wheatlets or the stuff shot out of cannons, or maybe crispies or crunchies — all of which hasn't contained a bit of life since it was emasculated in the processor's factory.

So far, if you have eaten any one or many of these — you haven't put one bit of living, decent food into your mouth or stomach.

If you think you can find health and long life in eating these dead foods — which, incidentally is the diet of most Canadians and Americans — then you are badly mistaken. That is why our doctors and other healers are so busy. That is why the pharmacists are busier than the one-armed paper hanger. That is why the drug houses are making millions and millions. That is why the hospitals are unable to handle the traffic.

You don't believe me? Well, you will, if you are lucky enough to survive long enough!

## MORE TO $H_2O$

Yes, there's more to natural water than meets the eye. Why do people and scientists run helter skelter everywhere in creation, it seems, seeking ways and means of procuring or bringing back health for themselves and others when the solution, the aid, the help is right before them ... metaphorically, an arm's length away?

While the great healers of the world are innoculating you with this, hypodermicizing you with that, tranquilizing you with another, immunizing you with something else — besides giving you a few dozen pills of different kinds and types for different purposes in between — the basic cause of your ill health is being ignored or forgotten. Nowadays they've got these fellows who are giving and taking synthetic drugs so mixed up that in order to keep you alive in the interim, they've got pills colored — pink, white, red, blue, brown, green and aquamarine, too, to match the green in your eyes. They make you swallow so many of the blue ones and so many of the pink ones, along with so many green ones. That's so that when they put the X-ray machine on you, your intestinal pipe fittings will show up in full color like a fancy juke box.

But to save all the hullabaloo and monkey-doodle business — if they just gave you back your plain, ordinary, natural water, you'd probably lose your aches and pains and be O.K. again. Yes, I mean the stuff that used to flow down the creeks and the streams and rivers in our country — the ones nowadays polluted by sewage.

Of course, if you told the medical officer of your city that you were drinking water from a stream, he'd say it's polluted and you're going to come down with typhoid or spinal meningitis or polio ... and he'd have you in quarantine so as not to infect the populace with the horrible disease germs with which you are polluted.

But hear me, hear me! The water that you drink in 99 communities out of 100 is at least chlorinated and in some places it is fluoridated.

The chlorination process simply kills most, if not all, of the living bacteria in water, and with the bacteria go the enzymes.

Yes, I do realize that most people will not concede — not even the scientists — that water contains enzymes. But

I say that water does contain enzymes, whether they like it or whether they lump it.

So the chlorination process kills all of the enzymes and most of the micro-organisms.

Now, did you know that plain, ordinary water as it flows from the creek or is brought up from the ground via a well contains many, yes, many vital minerals? Do you also know that rain water and distilled water contain none? (Except such gaseous elements that rain water picks up as it falls from the sky) That is why both distilled and rain water are known as soft water while lake, ocean and well water are called hard water. You see, the latter waters contain many minerals.

Well, when you drink natural water from a stream or from the well, you are getting your minerals and of course, you are getting the enzymes along with them to make those minerals available to your body. But after that selfsame water has been chlorinated or boiled or treated in other ways, the enzymes are no longer alive and while you drink the minerals, your body, in most cases, cannot utilize them ... and you are being cheated of a free meal and what is more important, free, abounding, joyful, good health.

If you have any doubts as to the veracity of my statement here, I ask you to go on a natural water drinking jag for a week or two and see the difference in your health and your well-being.


## MIRACLE FOODS

Most people throughout the world seem to believe that there are such things as miracle foods or wonder foods or better foods ... just as there are millions who believe in the existence of miracle drugs. Actually the term "miracle food" has no true significance or meaning from the viewpoint of a sensible nutritionist or scientist. It is recognized, however, that the term might have a different meaning or significance to different people.

During the years in which I have been studying food

and health I have been told and in some cases actually believed that many foods had the power to really perform miracles in regard to human health and in curing or conquering a disease. If you have been following the advertisements and the articles in many of the health magazines that are published in America and abroad, you will come across things like alfalfa, honey, queen bee food or royal jelly, yoghurt, brewer's yeast, bonemeal, safflower and corn and sunflower and other vegetable oils, blackstrap molasses, wheat germ, wheat germ oil, soya beans, sunflower seeds, soya milk, papayas, citrus, rice polishings and kindred products that are said to have miraculous healing qualities.

I must admit that I, too, believed and accepted these claims and consumed things like alfalfa, blackstrap molasses, cider vinegar and honey with a hope of gaining some material help healthwise.

Let me emphasize that most of these foods that I have mentioned are good foods — mighty good foods — but on the other hand, so are raw carrots, cabbage, avocados, apples, bananas, turnips, artichokes and oh, I could go on endlessly. My definite findings and studies have revealed that most naturally grown foods are valuable foods . . . that is, they have the ability to sustain and maintain health and long life in a human being.

Good, natural, organically grown food in wide variety leaves no great margin of choice regarding nutritive value. A pear is about as good as an apple. Nor is there much to choose between celery, lettuce and cabbage as far as food value is concerned. We need them all and many more for balanced nutrition.

It is also an accepted clear cut fact that if you eat the best of food and even eat it raw so that you will get its full nutritive value, but drink ten cups of coffee a day, with white sugar and cream, and smoke two packages of cigarettes a day, and drink a fairly good amount of liquor or beer . . . well, I'm afraid the good wholesome natural food, miracle or otherwise, can't do any more than stave off the cataclysm that is bound to strike you.

The best of foods can only perform their full functions as long as the individual does not destroy the body's integrity and ability to metabolize them.

So let it be understood that in my opinion you can call any food a miracle food if it contributes to one's health and well-being. But to fit into that class it must be wholesome, organically grown, unsprayed and uncontaminated. This would encompass fruits, grains, nuts and vegetables. I cannot, from my studies, include any animal foods in that esteemed group.

Now I will give you the real lowdown . . . and here is something of very great importance. All of the decent, uncooked, natural foods are miracle foods because they are, in truth, just that . . . for they are, if consumed in balance, capable of sustaining the body in perfect health. But there is no cooked or processed food that will in any degree fit into this exalted category — be it meat, fish, fowl, grain, nut, fruit or vegetable.

Strange to relate, my scrutiny and explorations indicate that grains, meat, fish and fowl seem to lose less of their nutrient value in cooking than do fruits and vegetables. As a rule, and it is only my opinion again, vegetables suffer the most from cooking — fruits next — and the grains seem to suffer the least. That is, the grains retain more food value when cooked than do vegetables and fruits.

For some time juices were heralded as performers of miracles — especially carrot juice. There were some people who carried the use of this juice to extremes and I daresay, some of them paid for it with their lives — which was clearly illustrated to me by the case of a man in my own home town.

A person with false teeth just can't chew the required quantity of vegetables such as cabbage or carrots. Well, for them a juicer is an absolute godsend and does greatly assist them in maintaining good health or regaining health that has been lost. Of course a blender might help retain all of the values by chopping up the contents of say an apple with a bit of water and then you could drink the

95

whole thing — it would be a sort of thick soup. However, it must be admitted that this is not nearly as palatable as the juice of an apple. One must admit that a freshly squeezed glass of apple juice tastes delectable and so do orange juice and carrot juice and pineapple juice.

There is very little that anyone can say if, for example, someone has found that the use of carrot juice has helped him over a difficult period or assisted him in regaining his health. And if he wants to call it a "miracle food," that is his or her privilege. But the same might conceivably hold true for bananas, papayas, mangos or celery or beets. Often it depends to a great extent upon the individual's viewpoint and personal preference. It is easy to understand that if one was suffering from a disease and the use of a certain kind of juice corrected the condition, then one might call that juice a miracle juice.

Fruit and vegetable juices have unqualifiedly proved their tremendous therapeutic value through the years and in thousands upon thousands of cases . . . and because of their fast beneficial action they come as close to being the true miracle food as anything else on earth.

For at least half a century milk has been lauded to the heavens as a miracle food and I have read a few authorities who claim that a human being could subsist on it in perfect health *ad infinitum* . . . but I presume these individuals have long since learned the idiocy of that statement. Milk was never meant or intended to be used as a food except for an infant or other newborn of any species. Milk was only intended by nature to be a means to an end . . . to suffice the newborn until such time as he or she could consume other foods — solid foods.

Skim milk and 2% milk are absolutely nothing but fragmented foods and they are not fit foods for a human being — especially for growing children who need all of the nutrients contained therein. The only way to obtain 100% of the nutrients in food is to use whole foods.

There are many packages of prepared so-called "miracle foods" on the market. Each one claims great potency and power for the product. Then, too, the bakery and some of the other industries claim that by fortifying their products they turn them into miracle foods that will perform great things for the human body, like building better bodies in twenty-seven different ways.

I feel that while one may have more, or less, virtue than another, still they are found wanting on the basis of performing any miracles. In fact, it has been proven that some of these so-called foods can cause harm to the human body.

I will again clearly state that there are no such things as miracle foods, but if miracles can be performed on sick, ailing and dying human bodies, that ability is found within natural, wholesome, fresh, uncooked or untreated fruits and vegetables.

Today I am quite convinced that a raw apple is just as good or just as much a miracle food as any so-called miracle food that was ever produced . . . and it will do as much or more for the body. A good variety of vegetables, fruits, nuts and grains in balance is the safest and surest way to good health and long life.

# CHAPTER 6

## Work and Rest

*"It seems difficult not to arrive at the conclusion that our motorized, mechanized 'effort saver' civilization is rapidly making us as soft as our processed foods, our foam-rubber mattresses and our balloon tires."*

. . . . JEAN MAYER, M.D.

### WORK AND LIVE

Are you waiting for retirement? Are you looking forward to the day when you can tell your boss to go to hell and hie yourself to your little cottage in the country, put your fanny on a chair and your feet on the table and say, "This is it!"

Well, I've got news for you, lad, news for you. If you do that, you won't live more than twelve, fifteen, eighteen or twenty-four months. That's exactly what happens to nine out of ten pensioners who take things easy.

I've learned that taking things easy at retirement is a surer killer than cancer or heart disease. Therefore, my warning and my advice to you is to get yourself a job or an occupation on retirement — keep yourself every bit as busy as you were before you retired. If you don't, you'll be sorry ... or at least your widow or your family will be.

I've learned that one of the safest and surest ways to a healthy and long life is through work and activity. Hard work never killed anybody, in spite of the fact that people drop dead of heart attacks when shovelling snow or climbing a hill or sawing wood. They would have dropped dead of a heart attack sooner if they didn't take this occasional bit of exercise. Had they taken more exercise and taken it steadily, they probably would have been alive yet.

### LEAVE LEISURE TO LIZARDS

You know that I am continually pointing out the dangers found in drugs and chemical additives in food, as well as the treated and fragmented foods. However, I would be remiss in my duties if I did not point out that there is a fairly high element of danger to be found in leisure.

Two men may consume identical foods, may commit identical sins (that is, biological sins against nature) yet one of them will come down with a heart attack and the other will take no harm. It would appear from the many studies and investigations that I have made, that sustained effort, exercise or manual labor seems to be an antidote for heart trouble.

Therefore, the added leisure that we have obtained through good labor laws or labor's efforts in general is in truth killing us. It appears that a human being was not made to sit around or laze about and do little or nothing. Every bit of evidence indicates that a human being was meant to work assiduously and, may I say unabashed, continuously.

Therefore, our greatest boon "leisure" turns out to be perhaps the greatest detriment to our health and welfare. So don't look forward to the time when you can retire and sit prone on your fanny because that may be akin to cashing in your chips.

## EXERCISE

It is right to refer to bodily exertion as exercise. And no one can deny that physical hard work is bodily exertion. Then what is the difference? My answer is that we usually get paid for work but exercise is fun and we do it willingly or even pay for the privilege of taking part in it . . . like golfing, curling and other forms of sport.

If you are going to do hard physical labor and be paid for it, and also gain good health thereby, I suggest that hard work is the greatest boon to civilization since the discovery of the wheel. Contrary to what most people believe, a man is indeed fortunate if he has a vocation that compels him to do a fair amount of physical labor.

Examining the evidence at hand, reading of the experiments conducted and also judging from my own personal experiences, I am convinced that exercise is probably the second most important factor in maintaining health. I try to make it clear that the first most important factor is food. If you don't have good, proper, decent food, then it is utterly impossible to maintain health ... and I claim that exercise is the second most valuable factor. In fact, the two run almost a dead heat in importance.

It is seldom if ever that a heart attack strikes a man who does physical labor. We all know that farmers are generally conceded to be a group of hard working individuals and anyone who has lived on a farm or been on a farm quickly recognizes this truism.

My studies reveal that a man can commit almost any non-physical or biological crime against his body, but as long as he has a fair to great amount of exercise and some good food he seems to be almost immune to the tragedies that befall men in sedentary employment.

It is recognized that athletes are not the longest lived among our occupational groups, which would tend to cancel out my theory. But here we are dealing with competitive athletics where the tendency is to over-strain and give the last ounce of energy that can be exerted by the body. This tends to strain and over-activity and no one would ever suggest that too much of anything is beneficial. There is a wide difference between constant regular physical effort and straining. Excesses, physical or mental, are to be positively avoided.

Furthermore, there is a strong tendency on the part of athletes, when they retire from competitive sports, to fall into occupations that do not require much activity. This sharp change in living pattern has its dangers ... for if they do not learn to curb their food habits, they often grow fat — which of course is a strong contributor to various disease-creating conditions.

If your occupation does not allow sufficient scope for exercise, there are various sports or hobbies which you can follow to give the body sufficient movement to maintain it in a healthy vigorous condition. One can indulge in walking, golfing, hiking, skiing ... and of course, one of the finest of all hobbies and a sure way to get adequate exercise for all the muscles of the body is gardening. It also pays excellent dividends. I would suggest that gardening is probably the foremost means of maintaining physical activity and good health. And if you undertake to become a gardener, the other forms of exercise are unnecessary. Yes, active gardening ranks superior to all for accrued benefits to the human body.

When I am asked why women live longer than men, I am quick to state what I believe to be the major reason ... women are usually much more active than men. And what is of even greater importance is the fact that this activity is continued long after most men have retired — taking it easy in a rocker and smoking a pipe. Women almost invariably have a longer working day than men and few women ever retire as most men do. A woman's work is never done. She has to prepare meals and do the household chores every day as long as she lives ... and that, I submit, is one of the chief reasons why women, as statistics reveal, outlive men. And according to the latest statistical figures, the margin of years is growing continually in favor of women.

Here is a bit of valuable advice for those of you who have not been active but who now realize the importance and value of exercise. Don't start into a great physical exercise program suddenly. Start with short walks or a few minutes devoted to exercise or gardening. Then gradually but deliberately increase the time factor and the pace of activity ... be it gardening, walking, running or any other form of exercise.

I specifically warn against sudden outbursts of physical energy. Don't all of a sudden decide that you're going to play baseball or football or you're going to do eighteen holes of golf if you haven't golfed for months or years. That is a good way to give yourself a heart attack.

It has long been recognized that good long walks at a good pace are most beneficial to people who suffer from constipation. If you are suffering on this account, I would suggest taking a long, smartly paced walk prior to the time you would attempt a bowel movement.

The medical profession is at last learning that lying in bed, completely inactive, is not best for heart and other illnesses. For the life of me I could never see why anyone would be put to complete rest in bed, as this can do nothing else but cause a slow but definite deterioration of organs and body tissues. I can, to some degree, understand a rest for people on long fasts, but for heart cases, who are being put to bed and fed, this only aggravates the heart condition . . . because the cholesterol intake is maintained without the exercise to wear down the cholesterol that has been built up.

I have pointed out that proper food is vital if one would enjoy optimum health . . . and so are good air, a decent pattern of living and a good mental attitude. But all of the best eating and nutritional habits on earth would be of little avail without physical exertion or exercise.

I have known many people in my lifetime who have violated practically every principle and code of living, yet they survived until ripe old age. I attribute this longevity in spite of the excesses to the fact that in every case they worked hard — they exerted themselves physically much more than the average man.

One of the big reasons why men who do hard physical work seldom fall ill in spite of bad eating and living habits is that exercise stimulates and activates their powers of elimination. They are able to excrete, through sweat, urine, faeces and other ways, many poisonous harmful toxins — especially the urogenic ones that would normally not be excreted. This is, in my opinion, the great benefit of heavy regular sustained physical effort. The persistent accelerated functioning of all parts of the body preserves the integrity of the organs.

On a recent visit to New Zealand I met a successful doctor who told me that in his many years of medical practice he never saw a hard-working man come down with a heart attack. It appears that somehow, by factors

102

not yet understood or discovered, hard work or strenuous exercise brings down the cholesterol level.

Now I do not suggest that you start working hard all of a sudden to lower your cholesterol level, because from recent experiments I have learned that it takes at least six months of strenuous exercising (starting slowly and gradually increasing the physical effort) to lower the blood serum level of the body. It appears that all muscles must be used and the accelerated blood flow performs some sort of miracle that removes the harmful cholesterol build-up from the arteries and the bloodstream.

The best advice that can be given to anyone is not to seek to make things too easy or too comfortable for yourself. Don't avoid bending or stooping or walking or running or lifting. Do your share or more than your share — within reason. Don't sit when you can walk. Work whenever the opportunity presents itself ... and if it doesn't present itself, create some. One can always find something to do. Maintain constant activity. Never sit or lounge about for long periods.

The entire range of all bodily functions, including each and every organ, can only function at its highest peak — yes, even with the best of food and water and air — if it is assisted by regular and efficient physical activity.

Here I'd like to quote from Dr. Robert G. Jackson, M.D.: "This is as it must be by reason of the physiological law 'that all cells, organs or body parts increase in functioning power the more they function up to, but never beyond, that point where exhaustion begins'; and also by reason of the other law that 'all unused, under-used, impeded or interfered-with cells, organs or body parts, tend to be destroyed'."

In "The Physiology of Muscular Exercise", Professor Bainbridge states: "The real value of exercise probably lies mainly in its effect upon the metabolism of the tissues themselves, and the vascular) changes are useful chiefly insofar as they assist more active metabolism. The speeding up of the metabolic activity of the body, which is a characteristic feature of exercise, involves the more rapid

103

utilization of reserve nutritive material and probably also the more complete oxidation of these materials within the cells. In this way it prevents the cells from being clogged with substances awaiting combustion, or with waste products awaiting removal, and enables the lamp of life to burn more brightly."

And Professor T. M. Tyler in "Gowth and Education" says: "The muscular system is the strategic centre, so to speak, from and through which we can reach, exercise and strengthen the intestines, lungs, kidneys, and all the organs essential to life, but which are beyond the direct control of the will. Hence the sturdy vigour of our ancestors and the dangers of a sedentary life."

## IMPORTANCE OF ACTIVITY

Anyone who has read my writings will no doubt have learned that I have stressed the value of proper diet in health. In fact, I have for some years pressed its importance more than any other single fact or principle. And while I will not back down on my firm conviction and belief, I also must accept the truth that physical labor or exercise is equally important in the prevention of most physical impairments and diseases.

The reason I am compelled to add this corollary is because I have through my lifetime known hundreds, yes, absolutely hundreds of men and women who violated practically every biological law and yet they remained in comparatively good health and lived to a normal or ripe old age. But in every one of these cases they indulged in strenuous exercise or hard labor all their lives. It could have been in the kitchen or the cellar, the barn or the ballroom, on walks in the country or on the hard city pavements ... but burn up energy they did.

I am forced to conclude that exercise dispels the harm of most bad health habits. There is no form of physical labor or exercise that I know of that does not promote better or improved breathing.

While we are discussing the matter of exercise and hard physical labor, it is wise to follow this rule. Prior to taking part in exercise or hard work, make sure that the stomach is empty, or at least is not over-stuffed, and the urine and the faecal matter are expelled. You don't have to be a genius to see the wisdom of that axiom.

It is advisable never to exercise or do extremely hard work in extremes of weather — be it too hot or too cold.

You see, we must realize the sober fact that hard work is something which is unknown to 90% or more of our population. Let's face it, hard physical labor is a thing of the past, especially in America. Therefore, we must resort to various forms of exercise to maintain our health.

Then one might ask, "When is it advisable to do one's exercises?"

My studies would reveal that upon rising in the morning is the best time for one's bodily exertions. But remember this, the selfsame exercise that is beneficial before eating is just as harmful immediately after eating. You might note that farmers do most of their heavy chores before breakfast... and farmers are healthier and live longer than most segments of our society.

Now while we are on the topic of exercise, remember this! Avoid exertion or violent movement of any kind following sex, eating or bathing. This warning is especially applicable to those who have any form of hypertension or a semblance of a heart condition. Also, never bathe, exercise or partake of any labor or indulge in sex immediately after eating.

I have always found that a good walk — not brisk or hurried — is most advisable after eating. On the other hand, if you prefer to rest, I can see no harm in it... but I think walking might be better. I would definitely advise resting in a supine position — that is, stretched out — not sitting curled or twisted up in a comfortable chair, for by curling up in a comfortable chair you are positively hampering the digestive organs in their work as well as preventing normal body functions.

105

Is sleep good? Is a lot of sleep better than not so much sleep? How many hours of sleep does a man require? Do you suggest six hours, eight hours, ten hours or twelve hours?

They tell me that young infants are best when they sleep most of the day. It is also believed that oldsters need more sleep than they did when they were young. On the other hand, I meet people who tell me that older folks need less sleep than when they were young. Then again someone else claims that the more active you are, the more sleep you require or should I say, the harder you work, the more sleep you require. Others say, the more you think, the more you use your brain, the more sleep you require. Then I find friends and acquaintances with whom I discussed this who claim exactly the opposite, that the harder working people, the hard thinking people, don't need very much sleep

So where are we?

Now let me give the benefits, good or bad, of my observations regarding sleep. First, I recall mother telling us when I was a youngster that sleep is a thief and if you let it, it will steal your life away. In those days as a boy I liked sleep and I'd never get up unless I was practically dragged out of bed or unless someone poured a glass of cold water over me.

I truly believed, as we are all taught, that you needed at least eight hours sleep a day. I haven't averaged eight hours sleep a day in the past twenty years. Within the last ten years I haven't averaged six hours sleep a day. At this stage of the game I submit that I don't get much over five hours sleep a day. And I'll say this . . . I don't feel tired or listless. I have all the energy that any one man can stand and I believe I am as alert as most people. I spend my days reading, working, writing, walking, talking, doing a few chores and I keep going usually from seven o'clock in the morning until after two o'clock in the morning . . . but I do get an hour's sleep somewhere between seven and eight-thirty in the evening.

# CHAPTER 7

## The Hunza Trail

*"It is of interest to note that the diets of the primitive groups which have shown a very high immunity to dental caries and freedom from other degenerative processes have all provided a nutrition containing at least four times these minimum requirements: whereas the displacing nutrition of commerce, consisting largely of white-flour products, sugar, polished rice, jams, canned goods and processed fats have invariably failed to provide even minimum requirements."*

. . . . DR. WESTON PRICE

### THE LESSON OF HUNZA

It was my good fortune to make an extended trip to Hunza in 1959. I went back again just to put my foot on Hunza soil in 1961. In 1963 I again went up to Baltit to visit my good friend, Mohamed Jamal Khan, the Mir of Hunza, to further investigate and explode or corroborate my previous findings.

I am most happy to report that the Hunzans are still the healthiest people on earth. I have travelled three times around the globe and made a fourth trip through most of Europe and I stoutly maintain that if there are healthier people anywhere, I have yet to find them.

For 2000 years the people of Hunza have been recognized as the best fighters, the most virile, the most energetic and the most durable of all of the peoples in that part of the world. They are feared and respected even today. When the people of Hunza migrate to other areas they are quickly recognized as leaders and are superior and make faster headway than any other people.

I was not the first to learn of the exceptionally fine health of these people. It was Sir Robert McCarrison, back at the turn of the century, who made this discovery. He had spent most of his life in India and the surrounding territory and he discovered the remarkable health of the Hunzans. So he went to the trouble of making investigations concerning their diet. He compared the diet of the Hunzans with that of the average Indian and with that of the British people.

Then he conducted some experiments. He fed rats on these three respective diets — Hunzan, Indian and British. The conclusive evidence proved that the rats on the Hunzan diet thrived and lived their full life span while the others died early.

I want to outline here what I believe to be the reasons for the good health of the people of Hunza.

First and foremost, the diet of the Hunza people is, in my opinion, largely responsible for their good health. They eat mostly raw foods ... not because they want it that way but because fuel is very scarce and they cannot afford to waste their fuel on cooking their food. The bit of wood that they do manage to procure is needed for heating their homes during the cold winter months. And in order to conserve the heat from this fuel, they do not have chimneys but only a hole in the roof. This hole has an adjustable cover over it to allow the smoke to escape when it gets too acrid and overpowering for them to bear.

Their breakfast consists almost entirely of a mixture of dried apricots, grain meal and their glacial water. They rub the wet apricots in the water between their hands and make a sort of gruel. To this they add freshly ground whole wheat, buckwheat, oats or barley meal and this is drunk like a soup.

Apricots, both dried and fresh, form a vital part of their food supply and the apricot kernels are stored until utilized — either eaten as nuts or used for making oil. This oil is made by each individual householder and it is made as required. This permits no rancidity or deterioration and none of the important nutritive values are removed. It is neither filtered nor strained.

They consume many varieties of raw vegetables — onions, potatoes, peas, beans, carrots, turnips, lettuce, radishes and others. There are many English walnut trees scattered throughout the country ... but the apricot is the mainstay. Too, they have grains like wheat, buckwheat, millet, rye, barley and some rice. They eat meat only on festive occasions, perhaps three or four times a year. They cannot afford to raise cattle for food since pasturelands are extremely scarce. They do drink some wine and practically every home has its little vineyard — that is, a few grape-vines strung along a wall or against the house. They do use butter or as they call it, ghee, which is made by heating the butter. Then it seems to spread better and keep better — at least, for their purposes.

Activity and physical exertion are the rules of the land ... by nature, not by law. The country in which they live is probably the most mountainous of any region on the face of the earth. They have very little flat tableland and therefore, they are always going either up or down. As wheeled vehicles, with the exception of the Mir's jeep, are non-existent and horses are few, walking is the rule and if loads are to be transported, they must be carried on their backs.

There are practically no fat people in Hunza — not even stout ones. The Mir was a little heavy in 1959, but today he is slender and fit. The Mir's brother, Ayesh, was the only stout man I saw in Hunza, but they do not eat the food of the ordinary people.

Very few individuals lead a sedentary life in that land. When they have grain to be ground into flour it must be carried to the mill and then carried back again. Every bit of wood must be brought from distant areas or from high up in the mountains. Their fodder for the cattle must be sought out from almost inaccessible bits of growing grass patches that are found here and there.

I have seen them risk their lives to obtain a bit of grass for their animals and then transport it back wrapped in a large blanket-like carrying apparatus over their shoulder. Every bit of food, fodder or fuel is come by the hard way. Everybody works and walks and everybody is healthy.

Another important contribution to their good health is their water. Their chief water supply comes from the Ultar Glacier — channelled to them by means of a conduit running most of the length of their country. It is a murky mud-grey in color. Laboratory research and studies reveal that this glacial water contains many minerals in colloid form, which means that they can be utilized by the human body. Thus, they derive many essential elements just by drinking this water.

No chemicals are used, be it for fertilizing their soil, for sprays or dusts or in their food. These harmful items have yet to find their way into Hunza. Their Mir claims that he will never allow them in . . . but time will tell.

In Hunza they lack most of the comforts of civilization as we know it. Only the Mir's palace boasts of electricity — supplied by a Diesel unit with oil brought in from Rawalpindi via Gilgit. They have no refrigerators, no labor-saving gadgets, no televisions or radios, no running hot and cold water, no motorized farm equipment or motor cars.

Their homes definitely lack the conveniences and comforts that we possess. This probably encourages them to spend most of their time outdoors, when weather permits.

Some of the Hunza men do smoke but these are mostly men who were once in the Pakistan army and they picked up the habit there and brought it back with them. Some of the younger men have tried to adopt the habit but it is discouraged. I did not see one cigar, cigarette or pipe lit by anyone while I was in Hunza — except by the Mir who smokes in his palace.

I learned that the incidence of infant mortality is quite high, but once they get past their infancy they seem to live long, healthy, vigorous lives. They do not have any of the hygienic advantages that we have in America, like toilet and bath facilities or even cooking or sleeping accommodations. In Hunza I found the homes quite clean and pleasant but they were certainly a far cry from even the most modest home in America.

I found no tooth brushes among the populace. Instead they use sticks cut from specific shrubs. They rub the ends of these sticks on their teeth and the fibres spread out like a brush and have a cleansing or burnishing effect. The teeth of the people of Hunza were excellent . . . in spite of some dental caries cropping up.

110

None of the degenerative and other diseases known in America are to be found in Hunza ... no cancer, no heart disease, no diabetes, no arthritis, no smallpox, no varicose veins, no renal disorders, no veneral diseases, no menopause troubles, no women's diseases, no hernia, no circulatory diseases. They did have one case of schizophrenia. (This information was gleaned from actual records.)

The chief afflictions of the people of Hunza are sore eyes, due to smoke in their houses, and intestinal disorders ... but they never develop into ulcers or cancer. The cause of these stomach disorders has yet to be explained.

The present doctor in Hunza recently arrived from East Pakistan and she wholly and enthusiastically corroborated my previous findings. On the occasions that I visited the hospital there were very few patients being treated. At that, most of them came from Nagir, on the opposite side of the river, and other neighboring principalities ... for this is the only medical centre in the entire area.

I established clearly by making investigations that the people of Hunza do live to be older than they do in other countries of the world. And it is true that the men of Hunza who are 60 and 70 and beyond look like our men of 40 and 50. There are only about 35,000 Hunzans and there are hundreds of them who are 70, 75, 80 and 90 years of age. The oldest man in Hunza was 108 years old when I visited them in 1963. I met him and he was still a good specimen of a man ... but his eyesight was failing.

There are other men and women who have been to Hunza but their stories differ somewhat from mine. One lady in particular tells the most fantastic fairy tales about their agility, strength and ages. According to her everybody or almost everybody in Hunza is 127, 140 or 160 years old. I repeat, investigation revealed that there is positively only one man in Hunza over 100 years of age.

The Hunza people are a healthy, happy, long-lived folk — an example for the rest of the world to watch and follow. Their way of life and their health are so good that

111

telling lies or exaggerating is like adding perfume and paint to a lovely red rose.

## YOUTH AND OLD AGE

I'm getting woefully weary because of the same old questions that people invariably ask of me.

"How does the standard of living in Hunza compare with that of the West and America?"

So help me, I'm as sure as fate that this question has been asked of me at least 150 times since I've returned from my travels in Hunza.

Invariably the people who ask this question are intelligent, capable people. Otherwise they wouldn't even know what Hunza was or where it was. So therefore I have to think before I reply. I don't dare say outwardly the things I want to say at the moment. I just stop for a moment and ponder and then . . . here is a resumé of what I usually say . . .

"Just exactly what do you mean by our standard of living? Is it television, motor cars, atomic energy, night clubs, movies or food you are talking about? Is it the style, the build, the type of houses we have, our libraries, our buildings, our roads, our hospitals, mental institutions or prisons? Just what do you refer to as our standard of living?"

One man said, "Well, I mean like where I came from we were lucky to get meat once a week, whereas in America if you want to eat meat three times a day, you can have it."

"Then," I said, "you are referring, strictly speaking, to the type or amount or quantity of food we can get here. Is that right?"

"Yes," he said, "I meant that!"

"Well, then," I replied, "you are not referring to a standard of living but to the standard of dying — because the food we eat is, as surely as the Lord made apples, killing us or definitely shortening our lives!

"There is something radically wrong with the way of life of people who are losing their ablest men at 40 and 50

112

years of age. Now in Hunza I can assure you that this is not the case.

"I remember three people in particular. One was Sherin Khan, another was Sultan Ali and the third was Shah Khan.

"I met Sherin Khan first. He was sent by the Mir to lead us across the difficult trails into Hunza. He was a soldier in the Pakistan army, on leave, who was going back home to Karimabad for this period. The Mir knew he was due for leave at this time and sent instructions ahead for him to join up with us and lead us through the Karakorums.

"As I sweated the first seventeen miles, at first through sand and later through tortuous climbs in the mountains, I was most uncomfortable, between the heat, the climbs and the altitude . . . and time after time I watched the soldier — his agility, his ease of pace, his gait and his simple, easy, quick, natural movements. He never showed even a faint sign of tiring, or any other difficulties through the sand, on the climbs or down the descents.

"Then I consoled myself by saying . . . well, after all, he's only a boy. I thought he was perhaps 19 — maybe 21. So bluntly I asked him his age and he told me 38. I almost fell over!

"Then I met Shah Khan at the Mir's. He was, strange to relate, the Mir's uncle . . . although much younger. He was probably the handsomest young man I'd met in many a moon . . . and his knowledge and experience amazed me. How, I thought to myself often, could a young boy know so much? I judged him to be not more than 18 years of age. And when in the company of young Jahangir Malik of Karachi whom I knew was 17, they looked as though they were the same age — boy companions.

"But a while back I recall reading Mrs. Lorimer's account of her stay in Hunza and in it she mentioned about meeting the handsomest boy that she had ever seen in her life and whom she called Little Lord Fauntleroy. She said he was the Mir's uncle — although much younger.

"It couldn't be — I thought to myself — it just couldn't

113

be! It's impossible. That would make him almost 40 years old, whereas this boy I saw couldn't be more than 18 or 19. But the evidence looked convincing, so I wrote the Mir when I returned home and asked him how old Shah Khan was. And the Mir obliged and said that he was 37 years old.

"Then there was Sultan Ali who was my guide on my walks and tours around Baltit, Karimabad, Aliabad and Altit. His pleasant, engaging smile and his carefree countenance made me suspect that perhaps he was 20 or 21 years of age — especially as he was a teacher. But out of curiosity I asked the Mir how old he was. And yes, he too was over 35.

"Outside of the old timer that I met who was 108 years old (or at least he said so) I never saw or met an old man in Hunza. I wondered about it . . . till I found out that all the young men were 60, 70 and 75. Up until 40 they look like boys. When they're 70, they look like we do when we're 45. Yes, some of the men that I met in Hunza who were 70 didn't even look 45 by our standards."

## HEALTHY HUNZAS

From the best information I have been able to gather, both from reading and on the scene, it seems that goitre was unknown in Hunza up until 25 or 30 years ago.

It is a fact that most of civilization's worst diseases are totally unknown in Hunza.

It was my good fortune to be able to visit Hunza on three occasions.

Now they have a doctor there who looks after the welfare of the people of Hunza and the neighboring state across the river, Nagir. The total population is between 40,000 and 50,000.

The doctor is not a busy man. He has a 10-bed hospital but only about two of the beds are usually occupied and he treats an average of two patients a day.

I engaged in conversation with Dr. Yussuf Mohammed Khan who was the resident doctor for that entire area when I was in Hunza on my first visit in 1959.

114

"Has there been any change in the physical condition of the people of this area?" I asked the doctor.

"Yes," he replied, "a little!"

"Do you regard them as the healthiest people in the world?" I asked him then.

He smiled and said, "Their health is undoubtedly much better than that of any people in this area."

"What changes in their health have you noticed, doctor?"

His answer was quick and ready. "I've noticed a high increase in the number of goitre cases and cavities in their teeth."

"To what do you attribute these conditions?"

"I do not know," was his answer.

"Well, how do you know that these conditions are on the increase?"

"Well, I have the records of the doctor who was here previously . . . although there has been no doctor here for a couple of years. Since the last one left they didn't seem to need one very badly. However, from the data that is available, I know that both goitre and caries of the teeth are on the increase."

"Have there been any noticeable changes in their way of life or the diet of the people?"

"I am unable to answer that question," the doctor replied, "because I have only been here for one year."

This discussion took place in the Mir's palace while being entertained by the Mir in his cozy, glassed-in living room that looked out on the most impressive mountain scenery that the world has to offer.

In a few minutes the Mir came over and sat with us.

"I've a problem," I said to him.

He looked concerned and said, "Can I help you?"

"Yes, you are just the man who can!"

"I am at your service," he replied.

"The doctor tells me that cases of goitre and cavities of the teeth are on the increase among your people."

"Yes, I know," the Mir quickly interjected. "I am kept informed."

115

"Do you know of anything that would cause this condition?"

"I have discussed that with the doctor," the Mir replied. "We see no reason for the increase in incidence of these diseases."

"Have there been any material changes in the way of living or in the food that your people eat that might account for the change?"

The Mir thought for a few minutes and then replied, "There have been some changes . . . but I have been doing all in my power to maintain our way of life and build a wall against outside influences. I have travelled, I have seen and nowhere are there healthier, longer lived people than my people."

"How right you are!" I echoed. "Is it true that up until ten years ago most of your few purchases came from the caravans that worked their way down from Kashgar?"

"Yes," he replied, "that is true."

"Is it not true, also, that now you get your supplies from Gilgit and that you are purchasing more from the outside world than you did formerly?"

"That, too, is correct," he answered.

"I read somewhere," I went on, "that the people of this area got their supply of salt from somewhere around Shimshal at the confluence of the Mustagh and Shimshal Rivers."

"Salt has been mined from that area for as long as our history dates back," he informed me.

"Where does your salt come from now?" I asked.

"It is brought in from Gilgit."

"Is there any difference between that salt and the salt you used to use?"

"Oh, there is a great difference," he said. "This salt is very much refined and pure, whereas the salt we got from Shimshal was crude and unrefined."

I sat for a minute or two without replying — looking from the doctor to the Mir and from the Mir back to the doctor.

"Do you see any connection?" I inquired of the doctor.

116

Then a surprised or enlightened look came over the doctor's face. "Why," he said, "I think you've got something!"

## HIGH-UP — FAT DOWN

Recently, through my searchings and readings, I came across something that put a little different slant on my investigations concerning the health of the people of Hunza.

It would appear that researchers have found that with people who live at the high altitudes meat and fat are not conducive to good health. This has something to do with the ability of the body to absorb required quantities of oxygen.

The report seems to indicate that where the diet is heavy in meat and fat the body requires greater quantities of oxygen for proper health. Therefore, it appears to be advisable to curtail the meat and fat ration in the diet of the people dwelling at the high altitudes.

Whether the people of Hunza have learned this bit of important knowledge or whether it is just an accident, I do not know. But it is unmistakable that suitable grazing grounds are few and far between in Hunza, with the result that widespread cattle raising is not feasible.

Therefore the food consumption of the people of Hunza is indeed low in meat and animal fats.

I do not attach reverberating importance to this announcement. I am just bringing it to light because it seems to tie in somehow with the fact that the people of Hunza are among the healthiest people in the world.

# CHAPTER 8

## Danger Ahead!

*"We start the day with caffeine, get through it with nicotine, relax in the evening with alcohol, start the next day with aspirin. Bubbling alkalizers remove yesterday's brown taste to make room for today's. That's the real trouble, and there's no pill for it."*
.... DR. ARTHUR H. STEINHAUS

## WHAT PRICE CIVILIZATION?

How about conducting a little experiment? You can have some fun, you can test your powers of observation and you can learn something.

Here it is. The next time you get into a bus, streetcar or a subway train, carefully appraise and examine the men and women or the boys and girls around you. Look at them carefully. With men and boys it will be easy because they're not covered with a thick paste of paint. See how many of them have the glow of health. See how many of them have skins that shine and eyes that sparkle. Inspect and examine and find out how many of them look alive, feel alive and are brimful of energy and pep. If it's in the morning, just look and see how many of them look beat even before the day begins.

Of course, with the female of the species you'll have more trouble, because you'll have to look beneath that coating I mentioned. But all the calcimine, paint and powder in creation can't give that vibrant tone to a skin and that bright and appealing glint to the eyes that nature in her kindness provides. Agreed, Michelangelo and Leonardo da Vinci learned how to create realistic figures, with even a gleam in the eye, but they never mastered the the art of creating within them pulsating life.

I'm telling you to do this scrutinizing business for your own enlightenment. I have gone through with it on many occasions and I was lucky if I could find two or three people in a whole busful or tramcarful that filled the bill healthwise. Is that the way it was intended?

118

Have you ever watched a squirrel fly from limb to limb in a tree — or even from tree to tree? Have you watched or heard a bird in the trees flutter and cavort about and sing? Or for that matter, have you carefully observed any form of wildlife in its native habitat? Do they resemble the humans, the people, the creatures that you see in a crowded bus or streetcar?

## A WORD TO THE WISE

If we are to listen to some of the vegetarians, or even those fellows or ladies who expound their beliefs in the raw food diet as being the only right way for man to live ... it would mean great consternation and sadness in our midst, because who among us doesn't enjoy the flavor, the taste and the pleasure of a good home cooked meal? I am the glutton of gluttons — and apart from that, I'm fond of food. Good food ... it moves me to ecstasy ... it makes me rant and rave and exude and bubble.

But no matter how delectable, delicious, irresistible, wonderful and marvelous foods are, one still has to think of one's health ... and the way to health is raw foods. From the records of the greatest food scientists in the world, I've gleaned that we need 50% raw, uncooked food in our daily diet to retain good health.

I'm not telling you what to do and I'm not trying to interfere with your way of living ... but I do seek to point out to you the way to health and long life. Whether or not you do it is strictly your own kettle of fish.

I would add to this, what better way is there to assist nature than by including in your diet as much natural food as possible?

How often have you heard a friend or acquaintance say, when he's over-indulging in something that he likes, "Oh, to heck with it! If I've got to worry about every bit of food I eat, and every time I take a drink ... to heck with it. I'd rather have a short life and a merry one."

Even a well-beloved brother of mine said the same thing to me on many occasions when I tapped him on the wrist to suggest that he was over-indulging. But he paid no heed — as millions of others pay no heed — but that won't stop me from trying. You see, I have a right to speak because I lost my brother a couple of years ago, and it was a sad loss to me because we were very close. Then I lost a sister, too, for more or less the same reason — human frailty.

## MOUNTAIN MOVERS

This is a sad tale . . . one that I don't particularly enjoy telling, but perhaps there is a lesson to be learned, and if that can help someone else, then it had best be told.

There was a lady working for me, and we'll call her Miss Schultz. She was in my employ for more than seven years. She was a faithful, diligent, steady person. One didn't notice her very much because she sat in one corner of the office and tended to her business. She seldom missed a day's work, and she was considered a steady, reliable employee.

Then, about a year ago, I noticed she wasn't present on all occasions, and then soon I found that she was going to Hamilton for treatments.

Don't ask how I knew, but I suspected cancer. Soon I heard that she was taking Cobalt or Radium treatments . . . then she was back to work again.

So, I went up one day and spoke to her, and talked to her about natural foods, nutrition, and such. It didn't make much of an impression; I could see that at a glance . . . So I asked her if I could lend her a book to read, and she said yes, she would take the book.

This was a small book about a lady doctor in Copenhagen, some quarter of a century ago, who had cancer of both breasts, and refused surgical treatment, and decided to cure herself and set up a health clinic . . . and she just died a couple of years ago at the ripe old age of 70-odd.

So I went down to my office, brought up this lady's book and gave it to Miss Schultz. Then after some time had elapsed, I asked her on various occasions if she had read the book or got anything out of it, and she said she hadn't had time, and eventually she brought the book back and I noticed, because of a little sleuthing habit of mine, that the book had never been read or even opened.

I am sort of a persevering guy, and I tried again, and suggested that she take some of our natural health foods home with her. Needless to say, she didn't. So, one day I went up to Natalie who is in charge of the department and said to her, "After I leave the office here, tell Miss Schultz she can have all of the natural health foods that she wants free, because I want her to try these natural foods."

The next day I asked my chief whether Miss Schultz had taken me up on my offer, and she said, "No, she turned it down flat. She said she didn't want it."

At this turn of events I was somewhat annoyed, though usually I am not as persistent as this ... but in this instance I spoke to her again about the importance of proper nutrition, and while I was speaking to her, I looked into her eyes, and never before had I seen quite the expression, or should I say contempt that poured from her eyes and face. I could just read it as though it were written bold and clear, and here is what it said, according to my imagination ...

"I am being doctored and treated by the finest medical men in the country; I am being looked after, nursed and guided in one of the best hospitals in Canada; I have the best nurses, the finest attendants, I have the most approved, highest quality medicines; I am shown every care and consideration by the entire hospital staff, and you, with your non-sensical books of trash, you poor, insignificant specimen of manhood, stand there and try to help me with your nasty, stupid, uncooked, unsterilized foods. Do you think that I'm crazy enough to pay any attention to you?"

So help me, I swear, that that is what the expression I saw in her eyes and face implied to me. I was beaten. I was humiliated. I turned around and left the office and her. I never spoke to her of health again.

A few days later she didn't turn up at work; my chief told me that she was in the hospital. She lay in the hospital for three months growing weaker and weaker ... but members of the staff who visited her reported back to me that she was in good spirits and had complete and absolute faith in her doctors and her attendants in the hospital.

A few weeks ago, a skeleton that was Miss Schultz was buried ... along with her indomitable faith.

## DETER — MENT TO HEALTH

Have we been blind or are we just ignoring the part that these new detergents are playing in our health and well-being? They have now become part and parcel of our mode of life and way of living.

That they are powerful, that they are effective for the purpose intended is proven ... but how harmful are they to our health? That is a moot question — one to which the answer will probably not be known for many years, because who is going to do the researching to prove that they are harmful? Surely not the manufacturers.

Today every dish, every pot, every pan and every knife, fork and spoon is washed in detergents. If they are so potent (and we know they are, for their own glib advertising tells us so) as to cause every bit of dirt or food remnants to vanish or disintegrate from our plates, then they must be respected for their potency.

Then why don't we realize that the residue of this chemical remains on our utensils and, therefore, is taken into our bodies with every mouthful of food we eat? Must we wait until many years have gone by and countless thousands have suffered and died from the effects of this deadly poison before we examine and see exactly what it is and what harm it does?

Most of our clothes today are washed in detergents and they are brought up against our bodies and contact our naked skin. Detergents are used when we take a bath, to soften the water. Again we are brought in contact with them on the surface of our bodies as well as in our mouths and stomachs.

Now it seems to me that ingredients that remove grease and dirt like magic could also remove bits or parts of our anatomy just as easily.

We must face the fact that the detergents are omnipresent and it should be clearly established by some individual or agency as to whether or not they are harmful.

## ABOUT COFFIN NAILS

It seems that all of a sudden a great emphasis or awareness has come up about smoking and cigarettes. Oh yes, they've positively linked them with lung cancer and heart attacks.

I have examined the evidence — stacks and stacks and stacks of it — and there isn't any doubt whatsoever that smoking is responsible for more than 95% of all the lung cancer cases and a large proportion of the cases of heart disease.

Now if you are one of those individuals who smokes and you like it and enjoy it and don't want to give it up and you want to kid yourself that what I'm saying is baloney, that's your privilege. But if you care to investigate and you want the truth, write to me and I'll submit it to you for your consideration . . . because there is no room for argument. The evidence is absolutely conclusive.

However, if you are a smoker, you may seek to defend the situation and you may say, "Why did this happen all of a sudden? Why didn't we know about these dangers ten, twenty, thirty or forty years ago?"

Now if you said that, you would be taking a rational approach to the problem and I would like it . . . because I respect people who think, ponder and question and don't accept anyone's word for the whole truth and gospel.

In my childhood I recall that people who smoked almost invariably rolled their own. There weren't too many tailormades sold fifty years ago . . . they were for the plutocrats. Yes, I go back to the days of the sack of Bull Durham when a man could almost roll a cigarette with one hand and handle a Colt 44 with the other. And

123

you'll recall that they had these rolled cigarettes dangling from their lips and quite frequently they'd go out and they'd practically need a box of matches with every cigarette.

Well, somehow I don't believe that smoking in those days was nearly as dangerous.

In the first place, you couldn't put too much tobacco in your cigarette in those days. Otherwise, it wouldn't roll or draw. Secondly, it would go out on you if you didn't keep drawing. Third, if you took the time to roll two packages a day, you'd be busy ... with the result that you didn't smoke as much.

Well, that's part of the story. But then you smoked only tobacco. Today they add saltpeter, syrup, sugar, dyes, coloring matter, flavoring, perfume and I don't know how many other things. It's not easy to find out either. Then, too, remember the heavy doses of killer sprays that are on the leaves and never removed, but go up in deadly fumes that you inhale as smoke. And for that there are no food laws or tolerances set up. In fact, I suspect that tobacco now is only a lesser or greater proportion of the thing they call a cigarette.

Whereas before you were only inhaling the smoke or the end result of burning tobacco, now you are inhaling saltpeter plus many other chemicals and additives that are contained within your cigarette. Further, I contend that all of these ingredients when they go up in smoke are more dangerous and more harmful to your body than the tobacco itself. But let it be clearly understood that I am not defending smoking.

Although I do admit that it can be pleasurable, soothing and satisfying, there isn't a shadow of doubt about it and no one can deny it — not even the presidents of the various tobacco companies — that cigarette smoking is positively harmful and deadly.

Part of the reason for the treatment of tobacco is of course to make the cigarette burn faster so that you smoke more of them and they'll have bigger sales. Then again, other additives help bring about the addiction. So here again . . . greed is at the root of the problem.

## I.Q. ON THE DECLINE

Here is something that is going to bring some name-calling down upon my head. I have a report from three friends of mine who are school teachers.

All three (each of whom I spoke to and questioned privately) claim that with each succeeding year the children in their classes become duller and duller. They maintain, (again, each one of them independently) that the I.Q. of the children in our schools is dropping drastically.

I checked this with a school principal and while he was not as emphatic, he did say enough to indicate that he found the intelligence of the children definitely not on the up-grade.

It is my contention that this condition is caused by the refinement in our food and the chemicals added to the foods. Or to say it bluntly and plainly, it is brought about by the defilement of our foods and the victims, it is tragic to say, are innocent unsuspecting children.

## HAVING TROUBLE WITH YOUR THROAT?

Of late and for some time previously, I've been asking questions of laymen and men on the street and many of the medical men of my acquaintance . . . Why are there so many complaints or difficulties with men's (or women's) throats and voices when they get around middle age?

Most of them gave the same reason in different forms . . . "Getting on in years" — "Old age creeping on" — "Throat muscles getting worn out". One rather alert medical man claimed that it was in the vocal organs that the first sign of bodily degeneration showed up.

One of the things to which I attribute the difficulty with one's vocal chords and throat is lack of exercise. When we were young we shouted, sang, yelped and hollered. The girls shrieked and screamed. But as youth faded, we shouted not at all and spoke less and sang rarely — perhaps only at a sing-song or in church. The sliding scale exercises of shouting and singing were missing and the muscles grew flabby and lost their snap.

Wait, there is another reason! Come with me behind the scenes and let me expostulate. Is there a man, woman or child among you who does not brush or clean his teeth? Besides, most of us who clean our teeth gargle our throats at the same time — using the abrasives, sands and other materials contained in these same toothpastes. Can you imagine what a rasping the poor, delicate membranes of our throats get at the hands of these miniature files?

You may ask why abrasives — why the moraine? I'll tell you why... Because if it didn't have that effect, it wouldn't be able to remove the film and accumulations of other matter and clean the teeth. Therefore, it wouldn't be used in tooth powders and toothpastes.

As a matter of fact, the more effective a toothpaste or powder is in cleaning and whitening the teeth, the more sure you can be that a greater abrasive action is used in the components of the mixture. All tooth powders and pastes may not contain abrasives in the form of sand, limestone or pumice. They may contain some type of acid or other chemical agents that act to remove the film or discoloration from teeth. But in all probability, this would be even more harmful on the tender fabrics of which the throat, larynx and other muscles are composed.

Could be you are one of the folks who clean their teeth after every meal which means at least three times a day... then maybe again on retiring and again on rising. Well, just imagine what it means to the throat to be gargled that often every day... or at least swished about with these harsh chemicals and abrasives.

I shamefully and sorrowfully admit to cleaning my teeth but once a day and that is in the morning. I think that's enough. You may not agree but that's your affair. You can clean yours as often as you like and scour off the enamel but I'll continue to clean mine once a day.

Just imagine the beating the poor, sensitive throat is getting — swishing all those abrasives and acids as well as pieces of this and that up against it, violently gargled and such! Why wouldn't the muscles give out or break down completely, for that matter? How are they to withstand such an onslaught continually, relentlessly?

It was just a few years ago that I had trouble with my throat and shamefully but quietly went to three different throat specialists. The first one told me there was some little thing down there that he thought he could fix and he gave me some powders to inhale. I didn't like the idea so I went to another doctor. He told me that there was nothing wrong with my throat. He could see a little inflammation but claimed it was just casual and would go away if I'd just stop talking so much.

A year later I went to another specialist and he said that he could see nothing wrong with my throat but he said he'd give me some medicine if I wanted it. I told him to keep it and use it on his polished brass.

After that I decided to look after my own needs, troubles and worries. In the first place I stopped using tooth powders or pastes of any kind. I use one thing — plain ordinary salt and I use it sparingly — just a few grains on the brush to give the once-over to my teeth. Incidentally my teeth are in good shape. I have 30 of the original 32 teeth in my mouth.

Secondly, I gargle only very, very slightly — just giving my throat a swish and out it comes. And I can tell you that I've felt a remarkable improvement in my throat. I think it's purely and simply because I don't give my throat the beating I used to give it.


## THE TRUTH ABOUT SUGAR

More than half a century ago, when I was just a lad, I heard stories that sugar was not good for my teeth, that it would cause decay and ultimate loss of my teeth. Actually the same story is still spread widely today in all parts of America.

At the time I didn't take this warning much to heart — any more than the boys and girls take it to heart today. A

127

the present time the sales of candy and pop and many other forms and ways of using sugar are more widespread than ever before in history.

Back about 1939 when World War II broke out and they began to ration sugar, I decided that I would forgo that tempting sweetening agent and live without it. And strange to say, I have lived without it . . . and believe it or not, I have my teeth, which I am sure I would not have had if I had continued my use of white sugar.

When I decided to give up white sugar, I wanted justification for my actions. So I did a bit of research on sugar. The general idea that I had of the way sugar harmed the teeth was that the sugar formed some sort of acid which found its way into crevices between the teeth and in some mysterious manner bored its way into the tooth and caused a cavity. But if this were the case, I reasoned, my teeth wouldn't decay if I swished some water around in my mouth. I tried this and it didn't work. Not even brushing three times a day helped — I still had cavities. So I made various thorough inquiries and found out the way sugar performs its dirty work.

When white sugar is taken into the body via the mouth, being almost wholly carbon, it cannot be readily assimilated or excreted by the body in its present form. Therefore, to eliminate it as quickly as possible, the body must combine it with other elements. Because the body recognizes the danger of sugar in the body, it will rob any part of the body to give sugar its needs so that it can be excreted. Therefore, the more sugar you use, the more vital nutrients your body will be forced to expropriate to get rid of the sugar. Thus, the nutrients that normally help maintain the integrity of your teeth are wasted and your teeth degenerate and decay. That is how sugar actually causes deterioration of the teeth. But let me tell you, it causes deterioration of other organs as well — make no mistake about it!

Now I'm not going to ask you to believe me or take my word for the fact that sugar is harmful. I want you to read this substantiated statement as it appeared in *Time*, January 13, 1958:

"*Sweet Tooth, Sour Facts*

"In the basement of Harvard's School of Dental Medicine, Biochemist James H. Shaw and his assistants worked for more than ten years with cages full of white rats and cotton rats, with sugar-rich and sugar-free chow, with test tubes and dissecting boards. The twofold aim: to find out how certain sugars promote tooth decay, then to find a way to forestall it. The Sugar Research Foundation, Inc., set up by the sugar industry, bankrolled the project for a total of $57,000. Now, in the Journal of the American Dental Association, Dr. Shaw reports his findings:

"Tooth decay is caused only by food remaining in the mouth — proved by feeding rats through stomach tubes. Even sugar, fed this way, causes no decay.

"Sugar, in solution, causes little decay; granulated sugar (as sprinkled on fruits and cereals) causes much more.

"Of the various kinds of sugar, fructose (from most fruit), glucose (from grapes and starch foods), sucrose (table sugar from cane or beets), lactose (from milk) and maltose (from beer) are all precipitators of decay. So is a high-starch diet, even when relatively low in sugar. It does no good to substitute raw for refined sugar, but blackstrap molasses causes a marked reduction in cavities.

"Saliva is a good tooth protector. Removal of successive salivary glands gave a progressive increase in decay.

"Penicillin and chlortetracycline (Aureomycin) are effective anti-decay agents, as are urea and dibasic ammonium carbonate; other antibiotics and chemicals tested (among them, many of those now commonly blended into toothpastes) do little or no good.

"Dr. Shaw's conclusion: 'We should cut down on our sugar consumption, particularly candy. We should be careful about sugar in forms that remain in the mouth because of their physical properties.' Along with his findings, Dr. Shaw also reported that his work has stopped.

Reason: the Sugar Research Foundation withdrew its support."

## IS SALT NECESSARY?

I condemn the use of salt in the human diet. I sincerely urge that its use be avoided or very narrowly restricted. There is not one shred of scientific proof that the normal body requires added salt. All the salt that the human body can possibly use is found in proper food, which is the only kind that any person should eat.

I have taken the pains and the trouble to investigate medical claims that the human body needs salt for various functions . . . and the one most usually suggested is for the production of hydrochloric acid for our gastric juices. Close study of the subject reveals that the body is totally incapable of breaking down sodium chloride to gain free chlorine to create hydrochloric acid. Furthermore, normal body functions excrete all excess sodium chloride or salt by every means at its disposal as rapidly as possible . . . because salt is a very harmful irritant to all animal tissue.

The only clinical proof offered wherein the body requires added salt is when the biological functions are disrupted by some specific disease. A diseased body may indicate a need for sodium in some form and therefore, it is assumed that salt is the answer . . . but even in such cases the salt does more harm than good. Salt has never cured anything but meat or fish or pickles . . . and the body of man was not created for pickling.

I have no personal objection to the flavor of salt in food . . . in fact, I have always been extremely over-fond of salt. But a study of more than five years on the subject proved conclusively that the use of added salt in the diet of any creature is not only totally unnecessary but positively harmful.

I want to stress here and now that all the salt that the human body requires can be found in adequate quantities in fruits, grains, nuts and vegetables. Furthermore, when found as nature provided it, it is in an organic and assimilable form.

Sea salt and natural unrefined salt are obviously better products for human use than the refined, chemically-treated table salt. But neither sea salt nor crude salt or added salt in any form is required for normal body functions.

## SINS OF THE PARENTS

I have before me a full page advertisement from a health magazine of February, 1962. In it is shown a child and a woman standing alongside a well designed machine and the caption above says, "For children's sake, fluoridated water in the home is available now with a home fluoridator."

Now at last doctors, dentists, scientists, researchers, nurses, demagogues and others who believe in or are sold on fluoridation can have all the fluorides for themselves and their families that they desire.

I would even go so far as to suggest that the fluorides be provided out of state funds ... because I'm so happy that I don't have to drink the stuff from my tap. And as a token of my gratitude, I am quite willing to kick in with my tax money for them to have all the fluorides they want.

When men have reached this depth of ignorance, brain-washing or blindness that they would inject fluorine into drinking water, then I say they richly deserve all of the doubtful benefits that this halogen can give them.

If, in this present day and age, there are people who have not taken the trouble to fully investigate the value or harm of fluorides but have taken it at their doctor's, their dentist's, their scientist's, their nurse's, their politician's or someone else's word, then I say that they deserve a good big belly full of fluoride ... and the sooner they get it, the better for all concerned.

My profound regret is that innocent children, who had no choice or voice in the matter, are the ones who will suffer and pay the price of their parents' folly.

# CHAPTER 9

## Pathway to Disaster

*"Why should a patient swallow a poison because he is ill, or take that which would make a well man sick ? Such practice has neither philosophy or common sense to recommend it. In sickness the body is already loaded with impurities: that is why it is ill. By taking drug medicines more impurity is added thereby, and the case is further embarrassed and harder to cure."*

; . . . ELMER LEE, M.A., M.D.

## I SAID "DRUGGED"

When I was a boy about fifty years ago I adopted an image of a man whom I considered a great man, a real he-man, a fighter for right and justice and liberty. Probably you had a similar image. He was known then as "the rugged American." That fearless, handsome, masculine image was pretty well accepted throughout the world.

But what happened to him? You don't even hear the phrase used any more — in fact, I haven't for many years now. And I admit that I am sad that he no longer appears on the scene or even in my mind's eye. Then to top it off, I could weep after I read a couple of American magazines or listen to the radio or watch a television program, for I see clearly and distinctly that the great, the glorious, the wonderful rugged American has disappeared from the scene . . . and the whole world is the loser.

Today the United States swallows more pills every day than the rest of the world combined. If you don't believe me, well, try to prove me a liar. I dare you!

Yes, I regret sincerely to have to say it, but the beloved and respected rugged American of old has been displaced by the "drugged" American.

Sometimes when I hear someone preaching and spouting about the great advances that have been made by mankind, I think back to the words of Ingersoll who said, "We have made some advances . . . we have stopped eating each other!"

132

Aspirin is the curse of our modern civilization!

I realize that millions and millions of people throughout America and other parts of the world rely upon aspirin to save them from suffering — to save them from agonizing pain — to save them from discomfort and various annoyances — and also that parents, especially women, give aspirins to children to save them the annoyances of a child crying or whimpering, especially during the night.

Now, I don't believe you women really think you're doing your child a favor, or do you want to keep kidding yourself? You know that you're only giving it to the child to keep the child quiet and thus, not bother mother and dad.

But take heed! Let's be honest with one another. Do you think aspirin is doing you or your child or anyone else any good? Do you think it does anybody any good? No, you know and I know that it doesn't do a bit of good. We know it in our hearts and know it in our heads and we know it in our souls. It does harm and the harm it does has never been measured.

"But," you say, "it does give relief."

Then I counter and say, "On the other hand, you know what goes up must come down . . . that life is a matter of balanced compensation. It might relieve your pain but remember, at a price. What is the price? Neither you nor I nor anyone else knows."

But more and more aspirins are used than ever before . . . and there is more sickness than ever before. Is there any connection?

Another thing . . . The best that aspirin can do for you or anyone else is destroy, hide or cover up symptoms. If a small fire starts in your house, would you drop a curtain in front of it to hide it from your view or anyone else's? If there was a leak in your plumbing, would you put a screen in front of it to hide it? If there was gas escaping from one of your pipes, would you spray some perfume over it to hide the odor? Of course not! How ridiculous are these suggestions! But do you realize you're doing something much worse in disguising symptoms — warnings of a far more dangerous enemy... because in one case you know you might lose your furniture or your house, in the second you might escape with a little discomfort and in the other case you might get away with a bit of water on the floor or spoil the rug. But in this instance, in all probability it will cost you or your loved ones health and life... for not only does the aspirin cover, disguise and hide symptoms, but brings, after a period of accumulation, reactions of its own.

Yes, because the aspirin disguises, hides, confuses the indicators and signs that nature gives you, the end result is more frequent, more serious, longer lasting headaches and problems.

## FEARFUL EARFUL

Listen to this pronouncement. It is my claim that many, if not most, of the dairy cows from which we get our supply of milk in Canada and the United States are practically permanent invalids. Therefore, we are using milk from sick, ailing, unhealthy, if not diseased animals... with which we feed our children and ourselves.

The short but productive lives of these docile beasts will in itself bear out my contention.

Here I wish to establish clearly that I am not laying the blame at the door of the farmer. In fact, I don't know exactly where the blame lies. But I do know that it has much to do with the prescribed feeding and treatment of these beasts by government agencies.

I am referring to the broad and unrestricted use of adjuvants, antibiotics, hormones, tranquilizers, enzymes, as well as other injections and treatments, and sprays for prophylactic and therapeutic purposes that are continually being foisted, injected and spread upon these poor dumb but beneficial animals.

Could the use of milk from these sick and ailing beasts not account for many of the problems that are affecting the youth and the children of today?

# HOW DEAD CAN YOU BE?

Antibiotics have made quite a name for themselves and they are probably the most widely used drugs in the world today. It seems that everybody uses them and takes them ... from infants to doddering old men and women. They have become as common as aspirins.

Strange to relate, I consider every chemical taken into the body an antibiotic. Of course the chemical and drug boys will not agree with me but listen, nevertheless. You know that "bio" means life and "biotic" relating to life. And anybody knows that "anti" means against or opposite ... and the opposite of life is death. Well, the plain simple unvarnished truth is that an antibiotic is a killer of life. Let you who will deny what I say is true ... but I firmly maintain that antibiotic means "killer of life" or "destroyer of life."

Antibiotics are killers, and the chemical and drug men urge you to take these killers of life when you are ill or suffering from some malady ... with the hope that these killers will kill whatever it is that is causing your trouble. What a fond hope! They're just as apt or more apt to kill the benefactors of your body. And don't laugh or treat this matter lightly.

Whenever anyone takes an antibiotic he is taking into his body a destroyer of life ... and it does destroy life, even if it is only a little bit at a time. But keep on piling it up and it will do the job thoroughly and completely. Maybe when they lay you in your grave you'll reap consolation when someone who wishes to be kind remarks, "He is only a little bit dead!"

# CHAPTER 10

## Adulterated Foods

*"Nowhere in the world is food treated so badly before it is eaten as in the United States. Here it is raised by the use of artificial chemicals. In an all-out effort aimed at quantity, rather than quality, we do everything humanly possible to destroy the original character that the Creator provided and intended for the yield of the earth. Moreover, by the time most of our food reaches the consumer, it is too highly processed, refined and improperly preserved."*

.... DR. L. M. MORRISON

### ADDITIVES

The big question that is invariably asked by people when they are first attracted to the organic or natural food way of living is, "Are food additives necessary?"

If you asked this question of a processor, a chemical manufacturer or a distributor of such foods, the answer would be, "Of course they are necessary for our way of life and if we didn't have them we would starve to death."

Then there are those who are a little more restrained in their approach and they say, "If we didn't have these additives, many of the products now sold and appreciated and demanded by the American public would not be available."

With this latter statement I am in complete agreement. Many of the products, in fact, most of the processed products on the shelves of the supermarkets would not be there if it were not for the chemical additives. It must be added here that there are now on the shelves of the supermarkets *many* so-called foods that are heavily loaded with harmful chemicals. For example, the various baking powders, ready-mixed products to pop into the oven, margarines, packaged soups, white bread, pickles, TV dinners, ice cream, the colas and many other soft drinks, and hundreds of other products and many frozen foods. Thus the people who must have or need these commodities have no alternative but to accept the additives.

However, there are as many or more products on the

shelves of the supermarkets that contain additives which do not need to be there. That is, the product can be made just as well without an additive as with it. For example, soups, cereals, cakes, jams and jellies, biscuits, cookies, crackers, candy, ice cream, cottage and other cheeses, beer and many others.

At this point let's divide the food and additive business into foods that positively will not keep without some preservative and foods to which additives are added for many reasons other than preserving. Everyone knows that jams and jellies and fruits can be kept without additives ... but the fruit treated in this way loses its color. The producer, when making jams and jellies, seeks to make them attractive so he'll sell more ... and as a result, he adds artificial coloring. So the long chain begins.

Then they go along and in other foods they add artificial flavoring, stabilizers, emulsifiers, firming agents, buffers, color retainers, anti-oxidants, anti-browning agents, maturing agents, texturizers, bactericides, form stabilizers, thickening agents, stimulants, fungistats, alkalizers, anti-sticking agents, flavor dispersants, polishing agents, mould inhibitors, color fixatives, leavening agents, bulking agents, bleaching agents, dough conditioners, binding agents, humectants, anti-foaming agents, improvers and of course some others that I don't know about. These chemicals are invariably put into food products for other reasons than preserving.

In my opinion, the preservatives themselves do enough harm to the foods by destroying their nutrient value or making them unassimilable by the body. However, there is a more serious aspect. These preservatives destroy body enzymes and harm other essential body organisms. Then, too, the body usually accumulates these harmful chemical substances in the tissues — fat, lymph glands and other organs.

But if you enjoy the convenience and want to eat processed and packaged foods, then chemical additives may be essential because these chemicals kill all living organisms in the food and thus, no decay. Then they tell us that these chemical agents are added for the benefit of the consumer ... and that is the biggest lie ever told!

I have discussed additives with various men in the field of processing and chemistry. Many of these men with whom I have come in contact are employed by, or are the managers or executives of the respective processing or chemical corporations. They all scoffed at the thought that there is any harm in the foods that they produce and sell.

If you suggested to the bakers of bread or pies, cakes and pastries that the seventy or more chemical ingredients that go into their concoctions could undermine the health of the nation, why, they would howl you down with derision.

"Our products," they would say, "have the complete approval of the Food and Drug Administration and for the bit that we remove from the flour we more than compensate by the high quality enriching agents that we put in. For a person to believe that our products contain any harmful ingredients is but a figment of the imagination."

And that's the way it goes. Each group maintains that the infinitesimal drop of chemicals that they put into their individual product not only does not do you harm but some of them even claim that it does you good.

Now remember, you get some of these in the meat and poultry you eat, the cheese you eat (even cottage cheese), the beer, the ice cream, the candy, the packaged and canned soups, the crackers, the biscuits, the cookies, the juices you drink, the cereals, the buns and coffee cakes, your peanut butter, margarine, all oils and butter and your milk and your jellies and your jams, and practically every product that you buy that has passed through a processor's hands.

It is claimed by all processors that they never use chemical additives that have not been approved by the Food and Drug directorates and, therefore, they are absolutely safe and can do you no harm — only good. Well, I want to tell you this. Irrespective of the position of the processors, the Food and Drug Administration, the Department of National Health and Welfare, the medical profession or

138

any scientific group, the chemical additive was never made that did not do some harm to the human system.

Here I would also like to mention that many chemical additives and drugs used by processors and others in both Canada and the United States have never been properly tested or approved by the government agencies. From Appendix A5399 of the Congressional Record 1957, we learn that there were 257 chemical food additives being used in our foods that had never been satisfactorily tested.

### A List of Chemical Additives Found in Your Food on an Average Day

Here I am giving you a chart that shows what the various foods you eat contain so that you can see for yourself what you are getting when you buy processed foods . . .

*Juice*
   Benzoic Acid (preservative)
   Dimethyl polysiloxane (anti-foaming agent)
   Saccharine

*Cereal*
   Butylated hydroxyanisole (antioxidant)
   Sodium acetate (buffer)
   FD & C Red #2 (dye)
   FD & C Yellow #5 (dye)
   Aluminum ammonium sulfate (acid)

*Bread*
   Sodium diacetate (mold inhibitor)
   Monoglyceride (emulsifier)
   Potassium bromate (maturing agent)
   Aluminum phosphate (improver)
   Calcium phosphate monobasic (dough conditioner)
   Choromine T (flour bleach)
   Aluminum potassium sulfate
       (acid — baking powder ingredient)
   Ditertiary-butyl-para Cresol

*Buns or Coffee Cake*
   Calcium propionate (mold inhibitor)
   Diglycerides (emulsifier)
   Sodium alginate (stabilizer)

139

Potassium bromate (maturing agent)
Aluminum phosphate (improver)
Butyric acid (butter flavor)
Cinnamaldehyde (cinnamon flavor)
Aluminum Chloride (dough conditioner)
Chloramine T (flour bleach)
Aluminum potassium sulfate
   (acid — in baking powder)

*Margarine*
Sodium benzoate (preservative)
Butylated hydroxyanisole (antioxidant)
Monoisopropyl citrate (sequestrant)
FD & C Yellow #3 (coloring)
Diacetyl (butter flavoring)
Stearyl citrate (metal scavenger)
Synthetic Vitamin A and D
Mono and isopropyl citrate

*Butter*
Hydrogen peroxide (bleach)
FD & C Yellow #3 (coloring)
Nordihydroguaiaretic acid (antioxidant)
Magensium oxide

*Milk*
Hydrogen peroxide (bactericide)
Oat gum (antioxidant)

*Jelly or Jam*
Sodium benzoate (preservative)
Dimethyl polysiloxane (anti-foaming agent)
Methyl cellulose (thickening agent)
Malic acid (acid)
Sodium potassium tartrate (buffer)
FD & C Green #3 (coloring for mint flavors)
FD & C Yellow #2 (coloring for mint flavors)
FD & C Yellow #5
   (coloring for imitation strawberry)
Gum tragacanth (stabilizer)

*Soup*
Butylated hydroxyanisole (antioxidant)
Dimethyl polysiloxane (anti-foaming agent)

Citric acid (dispersant in soup base)
Sodium phosphate dibasic (emulsion for tomato soup)

*Crackers*
Butylated hydroxyanisole (antioxidant)
Aluminum bicarbonate (leavening agent)
Sodium bicarbonate (alkali)
Di-glyceride (emulsifying agent)
Methylcellulose (bulking agent in low calorie crackers)
Potassium bromate (maturing agent)
Chloramine T (flour bleach)

*Sandwiches*
Sodium diacetate (mold inhibitor)
Mono-glyceride (emulsifier)
Potassium bromate (maturing agent)
Aluminum phosphate (improver)
Calcium phosphate monobasic (dough conditioner)
Chloromine T (flour bleach)
Aluminum potassium sulfate
    (acid — baking powder ingredient)
Ascorbate (antioxidant)
Sodium or potassium nitrate (color fixative)
Sodium chloride (preservative)
Guar gum (binder)
Hydrogen peroxide (bleach)
FD & C Yellow #3 (coloring)
Nordihydroguaiaretic acid (antioxidant)

*Candy*
Sorbic acid (fungistat)
Butylated hydroxyanisole (antioxidant)
Mono- and Di-glycerides (emulsifying agents)
Polyoxyethylene (20) sorbitan monolaurate
    (flavor dispersant)
Sodium alginate (stabilizer)
Calcium carbonate (neutralizer)
Cinnamaldehyde (cinnamon flavoring)
Titanimoxide (white pigment)
Mannitol (anti-sticking agent)
Petrolatum (candy polish)
Propyleneglycol (mold inhibitor)

Calcium oxide (alkali)
Sodium citrate (buffer)
Sodium benzoate (preservative)

*Sodas and Soft Drinks (Pop)*
Sorbic acid (fungistat)
Sodium benzoate (preservative)
Polyoxyethylene (20) sorbitan monolaurate
   (flavor dispersant)
Sodium alginate (stabilizer)
FD & C Blue #1 (brilliant blue coloring)
FD & C Yellow #5 (coloring)
Cinnamaldehyde (cinnamon flavoring)
Caffeine (stimulant added to cola drinks)
Butylated hydroxyanisole (antioxidant)

*Ice Cream*
Mono- and di-glycerides (emulsifier)
Agar-agar (thickening agent)
Calcium carbonate (neutralizer)
Sodium citrate (buffer)
Amylacetate (banana flavoring)
Vanilldene kectone (imitation vanilla flavoring)
Hydrogen peroxide (bactericide)
Oat gum (antioxidant)
Carboxymethylcellulose

*Fruit Cocktail*
Calcium hypochlorite (germacide wash)
Sodium chloride (prevent browning)
Sodium hydroxide (peeling agent)
Calcium hydroxide (firming agent)
Sodium metasalicate
   (peeling solution for peaches)
Sorbic acid (fungistat)
Sulfur dioxide (preservative)
FD & C Red #3 (coloring for cherries)

*Meat*
Alkanate (dye)
Methylviolet (marking ink)
Asafoetida (onion flavoring)
Sodium nitrite (color fixative)

142

Sodium chloride (preservative)
Ascorbate (anti-oxidant)
Calcium phosphate (anti-caking agent)
Sodium ascorbate (antioxidant)
Guar gum (binder)
Sodium phosphate (buffer)
Sodium nitrate or Potassium nitrate (color fixatives)
Magnesium carbonate (drying agent)
Diethylstilbestrol
*Canned Peas*
Magnesium carbonate (alkali)
Magnesium chloride (color-retention and firming agent)
Sodium chloride (preservative)
*Fruit Pie*
Sodium diacetate (mold inhibitor)
Sorbic acid (fungistat)
Butylated hydroxyanisole (antioxidant)
Sodium sulfite (anti-browning)
Mono- and di-glycerides (emulsifier)
Aluminum ammonium sulfate (acid)
FD & C Red #3 (cherry coloring)
Calcium chloride (apple pie mix firming agent)
Sodium benzoate (mincemeat preservative)
Potassium bromate (maturing agent)
Chloromine T (flour bleach)
Pie will also contain additives found in shortening and
   white flour used in making the crust.
*Cottage Cheese*
Annatto (vegetable dye)
Cochineal (dye)
Diacetyl (butter flavoring,
Sodium hypochlorite (curd washing)
Hydrogen peroxide (preservative)
Calcined gypsum or hydrated calcium sulphate.
*Cheese (Processed)*
Calcium propionate (preservative)
Calcium citrate (plasticiser)
Sodium citrate (emulsifier)
Sodium phosphate (texturizer)

143

Sodium alginate (stabilizer)
Chloromine T (deodorant)
Acetic acid (acid)
FD & C Yellow #3 (coloring)
Aluminum potassium sulfate (firming agent)
Hydrogen peroxide (bactericide)
Pyroligneous acid (smoke flavor)

*Beer*

Potassium bi-sulfite (preservative)
Dextrim (foam stabilizer)
Hydrochloric acid (Adjustment to pH
Calcium sulfate (yeast food)
Magnesium sulfate (water corrective)
Polymixin B (antibiotic)

*Salt*

Magnesium carbonate (wet-proofing, anti-caking and
    conditioning agent)
Sodium thiosulphate
    (to prevent decomposition of the iodide)
Potassium iodide (iodine supplement)
Tricalcium phosphate (wet-proofing, anti-caking and
    conditioning agent)
Calcium aluminum silicate
    (wet-proofing, anti-caking and conditioning agent)
Hydrated calcium silicate
    (wet-proofing, anti-caking and conditioning agent)
Sodium aluminum silicate
    (wet-proofing, anti-caking and conditioning agent)

Lest anyone tell you that chemicals are essential and that
if we didn't have them we would starve to death, I would
suggest that they are expressing only their ignorance and
bigotedness and are rising to defend their high salaried
positions or the fat retainers that they receive. The world
existed for thousands of years without chemical additives
and great civilizations — as great and even greater than
our present civilization — have come and gone without
chemical additives. There are millions of people living in
the world today who do not use chemical additives...

and many in much better health than those who do use them.

It is my belief and conviction, based upon observation, study and scientific data, that much of our sickness and degeneration is due to the chemicals in our foods. As far as I can see the only people to benefit from the chemical additives are the processors and their employees, the hospitals, the medical and nursing professions and all people concerned with and employed in these various hospital schemes, as well as healers in general. To these people, and to these people only, chemical additives are a boon.

## UNBELIEVABLE BUT TRUE

I'm sure you all realize that most or all of your processed foods contain various chemicals which I claim unconditionally to be harmful. But perhaps you didn't know that canned foods also contain chemicals.

In fact, this came as rather a surprise to me some time ago. You see, I felt that canned foods were bad enough because they had the very devil cooked out of them and therefore were useless as a food . . . or at least, the nutrients contained in the food were no longer available to one's body . . . but I did not fully realize that they contained so many chemicals.

Now there are various reasons why these chemicals are added. You see, many things take place in the cooking and as most of them have to be cooked at a high temperature, many changes would take place. So these chemicals are added so that the changes will not take place to spoil the appearance, the color, the feel or the firmness of the fruit or vegetable.

Here I want to give you the names of some of the chemicals that are used in canning . . .

You've heard of calcium chloride, haven't you? It's the stuff that's used to melt snow and when it gets on your automobile it causes the metal parts to disintegrate. Well, it is a toxic chemical that does cause gastric irritation and renal impairment. That means it louses up your kidneys. It is used in the canning of milk to adjust the "salt balance" of the product and prevent it from curdling. It is generally found in your canned or evaporated milk. And that is an added feature you get without paying for it... a nice healthy dose of calcium chloride.

But there are other bargains you get in your evaporated milk! Often they put in sodium phosphate and sodium citrate. And if you happen to have either high blood pressure or some kidney trouble, well, you'll get a real kick that will necessitate doctor or hospital bills. But of course the canner won't charge you for this. Here is where your "standardization" loophole prevents you from knowing what goes into your canned milk.

Now just think of the mothers — the millions of mothers throughout America who are feeding their babies with canned milk, assuming that the product is 100% wholesome, free of preservatives and artificial flavoring.

Now let's go on to something else.

When you buy a can of white potatoes and take them out of the can, they are firm and white. But this firmness and whiteness is not natural. It is obtained by means of a chemical additive and it could be calcium chloride, calcium sulphate, calcium citrate or calcium phosphate ... and all of these chemicals do not do your body any good.

Now in the canning of peas they use chemicals to retain the original green color or enhance the original green color or prevent the breakdown of the natural chlorophyll. So prior to canning, the peas are usually treated with magnesia or magnesium carbonate. These chemicals are known as powerful laxatives, so you get a free intestinal house-cleaning for the same money — whether you like it or whether you don't. I might mention that these chemicals are also used in fire-proofing wood, in disinfectants and in the manufacture of cotton fabrics. And the only reason that you get the free intestinal cleaning is that this chemical is so harmful and undesirable and offensive to your body that it takes every means to expel it as quickly as possible.

When you buy shrimps or other sea foods, they contain

chemicals which do not have to be stated on the label. To begin with, they use a nice deadly poisonous acid dip to prevent subsequent discoloration of the fish meat. Usually it is diluted acetic acid or citric acid. They also use glassy polyphosphates. Acetic acid is widely used in the manufacture of plastics, in dying silks and as a caustic for removing warts.

I have good reason to know that the officials of the Food and Drug Administration privately dislike very much the exemption of "standardized" canned foods from labelling requirements and they also admit that it is undoubtedly and unqualifiedly a deception. But there is nothing they can do about it because the bigwigs in the processing industry got together with the bigwigs in the government and put the deal through... and thus the Food and Drug have nothing to do with it whatsoever.

## VEGETARIANS ACHTUNG

Do you use milk substitutes? If you do, don't!

I have given deep thought and study to the matter and I find that in practically every case — in fact, every case that I investigated — the substitution was far worse than milk.

Of course, raw milk is preferable ... that is, clean certified raw milk. But even pasteurized milk is much superior to either dried milk or dried milk powder, evaporated, condensed or sweetened canned milk, and of course, the worst of all are the milk substitutes ... be they soya milk or other.

Read the label, read what they are made from, and you will know that I speak the truth. For example, here is what appears on one of the labels.

"*Ingredients:* A Pasteurized Blend of Water, Hydrogenated Vegetable Oils, Dextrose, Soya Protein, Carrageen, Modified Vegetable Gum, Special (U) Mono & Diglycerides of the Fat Forming Acids (except Lauric), Special (U) Propylene Glycol Monostearate, Lecithin, Salt, Artificial color and Artificial flavor."

If the above were not dastardly enough, here are more

147

horrors that are used in the substitute milk products: vegetable shortening, dicalcium phosphate, calcium phosphate, potassium phosphate and hexane gas and its reactions that were used in the original soya beans to remove the oil.

So in case you think you are getting a wholesome product, believe me, you are being badly rooked. If you are a vegetarian attempting to avoid animal products, let me warn you that instead they are giving you a vile, vicious, harmful chemical product and you are being seriously harmed.

Watch out for milk substitutes!

## IT FIGURES, NO?

What does a preservative do to food, or how does it act so as to preserve the food?

Invariably the preservative has the power to destroy many, most, or all forms of bacteria and enzymes. I repeat . . . this preservative has the power to destroy many, most or all the bacteria and enzymes with which it comes in contact. But here's the rub — we eat the food containing the destroying angel.

But what makes you think or believe or suspect that the destroying angel, that preservative, has satisfied its murderous appetite?

It hasn't. It will continue to destroy your body bacteria and your body enzymes as well!

Is that too far-fetched, too hard to believe or accept? When you turn poison gas loose — remember, it won't only kill your enemies — it will kill your friends and you as well, if you get in its way.

Preservatives can't distinguish between your body enzymes and your body bacteria or the bacteria in the foods that it's supposed to kill.

Therefore, you see and understand that when a food contains a preservative — that preservative is a positive menace to your health in many ways.

Don't ever forget that! And what's even more important,

148

remember ... this preservative does not only destroy the bacteria and the enzymes, but probably every semblance of nutritional value in your food as well.

## SUGAR SWEET NOT A TREAT

Please pay careful attention to this article — it is vitally important to you and your family! If you have any doubts concerning the value of white sugar, read the article below ... carefully.

"In the *Los Angeles Times*, Dr. Phillip M. Lowell gives details, remarking that sugar is de-vitalized, demineralized, and robbed of its life-giving qualities. In the main, it is made today, not from cane, but from beet.

"Cut off tops and part of neck to remove minerals, aid crystallization. Beets then sliced, and the sugar dissolved in running water. It emerges jet black.

"To precipitate some of the 'impurities', lime or carbon dioxide is added. Juice is then centrifuged, separating into molasses and raw beet sugar.

"The sugar is then well heated — destroys all organic life-celled substance.

"Acid calcium, phosphate, phosphoric acid and milk of lime are then added.

"To remove proteins, blood albumen (mainly from pigs) is added. Then filtered through bone-black or animal charcoal (again mostly from hogs).

"Twice the sugar has been boiled; now a third time, to separate it from the syrup.

"Then bleached with a strong agent such as blue water.

"All this is for first-grade sugar. Inferior grades are extracted from molasses by calcium and barium hydroxide. The molasses is used in gelatine, jams and baking produce.

"Commercial sugar is 'the ultimate extreme in food degeneration ... the term food is a misnomer. Sugar is the most injurious product in our national dietary, with no exception and under every possible condition'."

## DEAD BREAD

When you buy the ordinary contaminated or useless

breads at the bakery or your supermarket or your grocery shop, always buy white bread. Never buy whole wheat or any of the other breads.

I can hear you screeching, "What?" and holding your head and making a mad dash towards me to try to strangle me.

But I calmly sit here in my easy chair and repeat, if you're going to buy that lifeless "staff", then buy white bread.

And now, I'll tell you why in simple, plain, understandable language.

Actual studies and experiments have revealed that it takes five times as much chemical poison to keep whole wheat bread from doing any of the many things that the bakers and the processors don't want it to do. I repeat, it takes five times as many poisonous chemicals to do the job as it does in white bread.

Therefore, isn't it logical, isn't it sensible, to use white bread if you are going to use either of those contaminated products?

Better you should use whole wheat bread properly baked or homemade, made from natural, untreated, unfragmented, fresh ground flour.

## IMPOTENCY IN YOUR MEAT

I've talked to you about diethylstilbestrol before. If you don't know what it is, it is a supposed hormone ... but I suggest that it is a synthetic drug that was used by the chicken-raisers and cattle-fatteners to give quick results in the raising of these animals.

Back about the time of the cranberry scare, the U.S. Food and Drug issued a directive forbidding the implanting of the chicken and the steer with these pellets in their throat and behind the ear.

All went well, or so I guess, for a very short time. But now they have found a new and better way of getting the diethylstilbestrol into the food supply of the nation and now it is surreptitiously put into the feed of the animals. This, of course, is a hundred times worse than the implant.

We'd have been better off if we'd left it alone. At least we weren't getting so much.

Now let me tell you something about diethylstilbestrol. Research reveals that it remains chiefly in the organ meats and in the tissues of the animals. Though the manufacturers and distributors of diethylstilbestrol will tell you that the product is excreted by the animals, I want to tell you that only a part is excreted. The rest goes into the animal's tissues and vital body parts.

I'd like to tell you that reports reveal that men working with diethylstilbestrol were feminized . . . yes, just by handling it, even when they wore prescribed clothing, including gloves and masks.

I have long contended that diethylstilbestrol produces diseased animals and these are used as food far and wide throughout America. Now the scientists won't go along and say or agree with me that the animals are diseased. They just phrase it by saying the tissue is abnormal.

It has been my contention for some years that the widespread use of diethylstilbestrol in animals that we use as food is causing a sexual derangement or degeneration of our people, especially our men. If your man is not what he used to be or what you think he ought to be, a check might reveal that he is getting good hefty doses of diethylstilbestrol in the fowl or the beef that he eats.

No, I am not advocating vegetarianism, but I do submit that good wholesome, natural, untreated, unpolluted, uncontaminated meat is better than that which is raised on diethylstilbestrol.

Oh, yes, I'd like to tell you what else diethylstilbestrol causes so I'll quote from the Merck Index:

"*Human Toxicity:* Large doses may cause anorexia, nausea, vomiting, abdominal pain, diarrhea, headache, dizziness, lethargy, paresthesia, skin eruptions, breast engorgement, uterine bleeding (including bleeding following withdrawal of drug), amenorrhea, loss of libido in males, dysuria, edema, congestive heart failure, mammary carcinoma in males. May cause or contribute to mammary or genital carcinoma in females. *Caution:* Hepatic disease.

151

Benign prostatic hypertrophy. History of mammary or genital carcinoma or familial history of these. Should not be employed for uterine bleeding unless possibility of carcinoma has been thoroughly investigated.

"*Vet. Use:* Chemical caponization of poultry."

## READ AND PLAY SAFE

When you buy foods, read the labels. The government does in some instances try to protect the general public. I say this in spite of the fact that I'm always pointing out and calling their attention to various neglects of one form or another.

When you see benzoate of soda or sodium benzoate marked on the label, don't eat that food. Sodium benzoate is a deadly poison in any quantity whether it is 1/10 of 1% or 1/20 of 1%. It does and must cause serious harm to your body functions.

Most pickles and many or most of the preserves, jams and jellies and other things do contain benzoate of soda. But the government of Canada makes it mandatory that when they use benzoate of soda, it must be printed on the label. So therefore, they are protecting you. Be wise enough to take advantage of that protection.

Let the manufacturers themselves eat the products that contain benzoate of soda.

## DON'T COMPLAIN — ACT!

When people tell me that they are helpless concerning the poisons or the harm or the additives in our foods, I am quick to point out to them that the statement they make is not true . . . they can help themselves if they will. John Q. Public can in a matter of days change the pattern of foods throughout America.

All they've got to do is stop buying white bread or bread with chemical additives. Or stop buying white sugar or other foods containing chemical additives. And in a matter of days or at the most, weeks the entire face of the situation would change. If these commodities — especially things like bread — were left on the shelves of the chain stores, you'd get action, Mr. & Mrs. John Q. Public, and get it quick.

But as long as you are willing to put up with it and pay good money for it, there is little or no chance of any change taking place.

Therefore, don't howl, don't squawk, don't jump and hoot and scream. You obviously like it the way it is because if you didn't like it, you'd stop buying it and change the whole works in a hurry.

Yes, there is a safe, sane, sure way to maintain your health. You can compel the processors to make the food that you want to eat. Just make it an absolute point to buy nothing with a chemical additive . . . be it fruit, vegetables, grains or nuts. Never buy dried fruits that have been treated with sulphur dioxide or other chemicals.

You hold the cure for the insidious malady right in your own hands. All you have to do is act!

# CHAPTER 11

## Is Fasting the Answer?

*"The human body has one ability not possessed by any machine — the ability to repair itself."*

ᵢᵢᵢᵢ GEORGE E. CRILE, JR., M.D.

### FASTING

The famed Plutarch wrote, "Instead of using medicine, rather fast a day."

First of all, let us define fasting.

According to the best knowledge that I could gather, it is the temporary abstinence from all food, and herein I want to emphasize that this does not include water. Fasting means the abstinence from all food. Another term, and one that is being widely accepted, is "physiological rest."

The purpose of the fast is to allow the body full range and scope to fulfil its self-healing functions to best advantage. The body is more capable of self-healing than any other force or forces on the face of the earth. Please allow me to emphasize that fasting in itself contributes absolutely nothing in a material way to the healing of the body, but it does permit the body to become 100% efficient in healing itself.

Fasting, under proper care or with adequate knowledge, is probably the surest and safest technique or means of regaining health ever conceived by the human mind. However, it must be recognized that fasting is useless and a waste of time and effort if the faster intends to or will return to his former way of life. I also wish to assert that if one intends to fast, it is impossible to predetermine the duration of the fast. This depends entirely upon one's physical condition or physical deterioration.

With many, a fast of three or four or five days is adequate to perform the function of returning the body to normal health. With others, it takes 20, 30, 40 or even 50 or 60 days. For one who has followed a lifetime of wrong living, along with the ingestion of various drugs, the system has become loaded with inorganic chemicals, drugs and synthetic chemical compounds and it cannot rid itself of these harmful, often caustic and searing foreign materials or their effects in the span of but a few days. This includes the so-called simple and supposedly harmless drugs. It will take weeks and sometimes even two months.

Records that I have examined have revealed that men and women have fasted up to sixty days with not only no perceptible harmful effects, but they have derived many benefits therefrom. Many or most of those who have taken long fasts express their enthusiasm in various ways but in summing it up, it would appear to be the closest thing to a panacea that they have ever encountered.

It is my sincere belief that fasting is the world's finest form of therapy. There is no doubt in my mind that the percentage of results obtained from fasting is higher than for any other form of healing. The results would be even greater and more dramatic if the person involved did not set out to fast after he found that he had one foot in the grave and the other on a banana peel. It is no exaggeration to say that people only come to a fast or start one or study about it when every other form of healing has been tried and found wanting. Yes, it is absolutely true that about 99 out of 100 people who fast do so only as a last resort. Therefore, because of this, it is virtually impossible to get 100% results.

I wish to stress that fasting is not the answer to every ailment or ache or pain or disease and it is wise to realize that for some ailments fasting can be seriously harmful. It is suggested that fasting not be undertaken for diseases such as hernia, chronic paralysis, advanced cancer (especially cancer of the liver), diabetes, lead poisoning, advanced osteo-arthritis and tuberculosis. However, upon close study benefits may be found even for these diseases ... but I stress, investigate thoroughly. And extreme caution should be taken in fasting by those who have had

155

recent surgery or where insulin has been used for more than two years.

At this time I would like to make a positive and definite distinction between starvation and fasting. They are in no way connected or related.

Starvation is denying the body essential food for its maintenance and is positively and definitely injurious and often fatal, whereas sensible fasting is temporary abstinence until the surplus or stored fats are consumed and harmful accumulations are eliminated and it is remedial, restorative and healthful.

Permit no one to promise you a cure, be it by fasting or any other means or method of therapy. Healing or curing is done by the body alone and thus, no one can speak for the individual human body. Its actions and reactions are governed strictly by itself and itself alone. However, the remarkable results achieved through fasting would indicate that it works and it permits nature to work at her best.

At the time this book is being written there are, according to my sources of information, less than ten experienced, qualified, non-medical fasting practitioners in all of America. However from my recent reading in the press and medical journals, I notice that medical doctors are beginning to use the art of fasting — and with top level success.

I have, in the course of my studies, come across a few incidences of death during fasts. These are comparatively rare but they do occur. My reaction, and that of many professional healers, is that the patient would have died at the same time or earlier anyway ... and fasting did not cause the death nor hurry it along.

It must be emphasized again and again that one should never attempt long fasts without the proper supervision or guidance. If one intends to undertake a fast on his own hook (which I do not advise) he should arm himself with sufficient knowledge ... and this takes time and effort! Never attempt it otherwise!

It appears that practically all the fields of healing are

doing some investigating (some serious, others cursory) concerning fasting — which is a rather good indication. It seems as though the various other healing professions suspect there is something to fasting. I understand that the Mayo Clinic at Rochester, Minnesota is having some research work done on fasting.

Here I quote Dr. Walter C. Alvarez, Emeritus Consultant in Medicine from the Mayo Clinic:

"In our experiments with animals my colleagues and I found that if we upset them by giving perhaps more fat than they could digest comfortably, for a few days afterward their digestion was poor, no matter what food we gave them. Then, the only way in which we could restore the animal to health was to give him no food for a couple of days."

Existing records would reveal that fasting is the oldest of all the healing processes ever practised by animals and humans. All animals practise fasting instinctively — man, only when he is truly enlightened.

Dr. Robert Walter says in "Life's Great Law":

"No process of treatment ever invented fulfils so many indications for restoration of health as does fasting. It is nature's own primal process, her first requirement in nearly all cases. As a means of promoting circulation, improving nutrition, facilitating excretion, recuperating vital power, and restoring vital vigor it has no competitor."

It has been positively and carefully observed that fasting causes the breakdown, absorption, dispersion, diffusion and elimination of abnormal growths as well as the egestion, extrusion, emanation and transudation of deposits and other afflictions.

It is an established fact that during fasting all the strictly mental powers of the human being are greatly sharpened and improved. The ability to reason is accelerated. Memory is toned up. Practically all of the sensory powers possessed by human beings are broadened and raised to a much higher level than normal during and after a fast.

From my interrogations, conversations and correspondence with men and women who have undergone long periods of fasting, and from studying their notes, it is clear that all of their intellectual powers, their intuition, understanding, sympathy and love and even sexual vigor were enhanced.

Here I'd like to quote from Dr. Henry S. Tanner, "It is evident that the prophets of old fasted for spiritual illumination. They must have derived some of their gifts or inspiration from their fasting."

While I make it clear and positive that fasting itself does not cure anything, I wish to point out some of the things that fasting does accomplish simply by enabling the organism to do what it needs to do for itself.

1. Gives overburdened organs rest and time for rehabilitation.
2. Sharpens and accentuates the mental faculties.
3. Improves the intestinal organs' ability to digest and assimilate food.
4. Conserves essential energy.
5. Promotes the breaking down, absorption and elimination of various abnormal growths and obstructions.
6. Allows the organs of elimination time to void accumulated matter.
7. Creates a feeling or condition of euphoria.
8. Makes the mind receptive to logic and sensible correct way of living.
9. Promotes the elimination of inorganic chemical accumulations that cannot be divested from the body by any other means.

While fasting is accepted and recognized as being the oldest form of therapy, it was Dr. Isaac Jennings, born in 1788 in Oberlin, Ohio, who was the first physician to advocate and use fasting in his treatment of the sick and ailing. He was an orthodox medical practitioner and after about ten years of practice he became convinced that fasting had merit. It is recorded that no one could compete with him when it came to being of help to the sick.

There are two other famous doctors who are credited with being the earliest of men to advocate and put the art of fasting into practice. They were Dr. Henry S. Tanner and Dr. Edward Hooker Dewey.

From studying much of the available material pertaining to fasting, it is clear to me that the body itself will indicate when the period of fasting should end and food once again be taken. Here it is important to draw a distinction between natural hunger and psychological hunger. Natural hunger takes place when all of the stores of fat and other accumulations have been used up or voided. When this occurs, the natural thing left for the body to do to prevent death from starvation is to begin to live off its own tissues. This would be most harmful. At this stage natural hunger occurs and food should be taken to prevent the body from feeding off itself.

It is at this point that the value of the practitioner is of vital importance. He is accustomed to recognizing the signs that indicate that the fast should be ended. It is also possible to learn for one's self the proper time to end a fast but it requires much reading, investigation, studying and general knowledge . . . and this is something that few individuals ever take the time to do. Therefore, it is advisable to be under the guidance or direction of a practitioner experienced in the art of fasting.

Now we list some experienced medical advice on the values of fasting:

*J. H. Tilden, M.D.* — "cases of pernicious anemia taken off their food will double their blood count in a week."

*George S. Weger, M.D.* — "hemoglobin increased 50 per cent and white cells were reduced 50 per cent on a twelve day fast."

*William Howard Hay, M.D.* — "101 pernicious anemia patients . . . only eight failed to recover."

*Hippocrates* — "The more you nourish a diseased body, the worse you make it."

*P. H. Dewey, M.D.* — "Take away food from a sick man's stomach and you have begun, not to starve the sick man, but the disease." "A fast starves, not the patient, but the disease."

*Hereward Carrington, Ph.D.* — "Therapeutic fasting is

159

based upon the now generally recognized fact that humanity is ill — as the hundreds of hospitals and thousands of doctors amply testify! Assuredly, something's wrong somewhere! All the evidence goes to show us that this state of affairs has been brought about largely by one simple factor: the majority of people eat too much food, and the wrong kind of food. Fasting rids the body of this surplus of toxic material, resting and purifying it at the same time. It is, so to say, merely a method of physiological housecleaning . . . Fasting is the greatest remedial agent in the world today. Its curative, purifying and therapeutic value is almost unlimited. It can restore health where all else fails. It is almost universally applicable. It is the greatest restorative and rejuvenator known to man. It is safe, economical and speedy. It can prolong life and prevent premature death. It is based upon sound physiology. What more could be asked of any 'cure'?"

*Alexis Carrel, M.D.*, one of the world's greatest scientists said: "The elimination of waste products by fasting increases longevity."

*Dr. Von Seeland*, of Russia, wrote, ". . . I have come to the conclusion that fasting is not only a therapeutic of the highest degree possible but also deserves consideration educationally."

*Prof. Child*, in his *Senescence and Rejuvenescence* remarks: "Partial starvation inhibits senescence. The starveling is brought back from an advanced age to the beginning of post-embryonic life; it is almost reborn."

## MORE ABOUT FASTING

I have been hearing about, reading about, studying and investigating fasting for almost fifteen years. Up until most recently I did not accept that form of therapy as being beneficial to the human body . . . that is, if it can be referred to as therapy. I find that I have been in error — in sad and great and tragic error. In fact, I may say that it is the most valuable type of therapy known to both man and beast.

I really can't tell you on what ground I opposed fasting except I didn't think it was natural. Then I learned that most animals do not eat when they are ill, that the ancient Biblical prophets fasted regularly, that Christ fasted for 40 days and that fasting has been practised for thousands of years. I have also learned that while on rare occasions someone may die of actual starvation, millions die because of the effects of just too much or improper food.

What convinced me that fasting has genuine merit was the many people whom I had met here, there and on my travels who told me that they had been brought back to life from the very gates of death, when all other means and methods had failed, simply by fasting.

The evidence became so overwhelming that I could no longer maintain my position. I had to bow. And then I began to dig and investigate, read and study. Today I think I know the reason why ... or would I say, reasons why.

I would not necessarily advocate fasting for a newborn infant ... although even this may prove to be of value, especially if the infant were suffering from any one of many conditions.

The strangest thing that I learned was that most of the so-called deficiency diseases known to man disappeared or were cleared up by fasting. This to me was a perfect paradox. How can you cause something to be filled by emptying it? Yet it is true — absolutely true!

Don't ask me why because I'm not sure that I can tell you. But here may be some of the reasons.

Certain foods, plus the chemical additives contained therein, must interfere with or prevent proper metabolism and assimilation. Now it could be true that the incorrect combinations of foods that a human being eats causes chemical imbalance ... and again it might be that over-abundance or too many harmful or wrong foods could be the culprit. But I have learned that it is absolutely true that one will find that many or most of the deficiency diseases, as well as many other diseases, disappear when a fast is undertaken.

161

Please don't run off with the idea that you can cure all diseases by fasting or that fasting is a cinch because if you do you will be making a serious mistake. Fasting has its place and in order to fast one should have proper supervision. Don't try any extended fasts alone . . . they can be dangerous!

# CHAPTER 12

## Enzymes: The Spark of Life

*"When you realize that each body cell is a small battery, needing constant recharging through the food you eat, you'll begin to really think about diet."*

    .... DR. J. D. NOLAN

### SECRET OF LIFE, HEALTH AND LIVING

I'm going to talk to you about enzymes. Those of you who have been interested in health for some time have obviously learned all about enzymes. But to most people — at least those whom I have met and encountered — enzyme is a word that they have heard but know little or nothing about.

From my knowledge and experience I have reached the conclusion that enzymes are the most important organisms in all the world. I might even go further and say that they are the most important things in all the world!

To me enzymes are symbols of life itself.

From here on I'm going to quote from a dictionary of biology published by Penguin Reference Books and it is written and compiled by M. Abercrombie, C. J. Hickman and M. L. Johnson. I am adding nothing and omitting nothing. But I ask you to study this lesson carefully because it can easily save your life ... and at least it may save you from illness.

In some places it is slightly technical. But even if you don't get the hang of the technical parts, you will get enough to make you understand why I stress the importance of untreated, natural, organic, uncontaminated, unpasteurized, unboiled, unfried and unbaked foods wherever humanly possible.

"ENZYME. A catalyst (i.e. a substance which in minute amounts promotes chemical change without itself being used up in the reaction), produced by living things, of complex structure. There are many different kinds, each kind acting only on a very limited range of chemical reactions.

"Within all living things a large number of chemical reactions are always in progress. The majority of these reactions are controlled by enzymes. An enzyme, like all catalysts, greatly increases the rate of chemical change of a substance or substances (called the substrate) to another or others. Most of the reactions of metabolism would not occur perceptibly in the absence of enzymes, at the temperature and in the other conditions in which living things exist; and so metabolism is entirely dependent on enzymes. An enzyme produces its effect on the substrate by combining with it and activating it, so that the substrate undergoes further chemical change, at the same time losing its combination with the enzyme. As the result of the process, therefore, the enzyme is not consumed, but at the end of the process is free to deal with more substrate. Since the activation of the substrate is rapid, a very small amount of enzyme can produce a very great effect. One molecule of catalase can decompose 40,000 molecules of hydrogen peroxide per second at freezing point. Most enzymes are in fact present in relatively minute amounts.

"Most enzymes activate only one kind of substrate each. Other enzymes are less highly specific but even so each reacts only with chemically related substrates. There is correspondingly a large number of different enzymes, for all the different reactions of metabolism.

"Each enzyme requires certain definite conditions for optimum performance, particularly as regards pH, the presence of specific accessory substances (co-enzymes, activators) and the absence of specific inhibiting substances.

"Enzymes are unstable substances, and are easily destroyed or inactivated, e.g. by high temperature, or by a great range of chemical substances. It is probable that, although they are not consumed by the reaction, enzymes slowly break down and have to be synthesized. The micronutrients required by organisms probably mostly go to regenerating enzymes and co-enzymes.

"Enzymes are all produced within living cells and most of them do their work there, though they can often be extracted and can be studied outside the cell. Some enzymes (e.g. digestive enzymes of vertebrates) are normally secreted to the outside of cells. In metabolic processes of cells, and also in digestion, enzymes work very much as systems, the products of one reaction passing on to be the substrate of another.

"Closely similar enzymes, and enzyme systems, have been found in a wide variety of organisms, including plants, animals, and bacteria, and they account for the fundamental similarities of many aspects of their metabolism.

"Several enzymes have been obtained pure and crystalline. Some of these are entirely protein; some are protein plus a prosthetic group."

## KEY TO LIFE

Enzymes are life. They are part and parcel of every living thing. No form of life can exist without them.

Therefore, it behooves you to know what they are and what they mean to you.

After delving into enzymes to a fair degree or depth, I find that very few people, including scientists, know much about this most unusual action . . . or should I say, form of life? Nobody knows what it is.

But the origin of the name will probably give you the closest clue as to how it can be classified. The name is derived from the Greek word "zyme" which means, to leaven . . . and it is the substance formed in or is part of living cells which promotes chemical change.

Now let me go further here and tell you that the enzyme level in the human body indicates disease or health. If you're loaded with enzymes, you're healthy and if you're depleted or low in them, you're sick.

I doubt if anyone has ever phrased it that way before — that is, that tersely — but I challenge anyone to show that this is not wholly true.

An alert, competent, well trained physician can detect various diseases by checking or studying the enzyme level of his patient.

You are probably quite aware of the fact that life begets

life. A dead plant that hasn't produced seed cannot propagate itself. If you consume living food, you can expect it to create and maintain a living body.

It is a fact that the human body is capable of synthesizing or creating enzymes of its own. But it is restricted in the type and kinds of enzymes that it can create. And as the enzyme intake of the body declines because of the incorrect food you eat, its enzyme-making abilities will also decline.

Now again I want to say that no one has yet correctly defined an enzyme. But they do know that enzymes are killed or rendered lifeless or inactive by heat, by radiation, by chemical gases, fumes and other things. Pasteurization kills them, chlorination kills them, flouridation kills them. They only remain alive and active if left alone, as nature intended.

The best authority that I could find claims that when you eat a banana, the part of the banana not assimilated, along with the enzymes originally found therein, passes out with the feces. It is just there to see that the job of the proper assimilation of food takes place.

But the ingestion of drugs or other harmful additives can and does inhibit or kill enzymes and that is how in many cases drugs do harm to the human body.

I've learned that some, many or all of the poison gases achieve their effect by killing your body enzymes. When enough of them are killed, then the human body can no longer function and death takes place.

## RIGHT TO THE POINT

Here I'm going to try to illustrate some of the functions, uses and purposes of enzymes in the natural order of things.

They are referred to as gastric ferments, also as digestive enzymes. Then, too, they form a part of your intestinal bacterial flora. In simple parlance, they are known as cleavage factors. They can also be called and are often referred to as splitting agents, which, by means of their chemical potency, break through the complex biochemical bonds of all natural, organic substances... especially our uncontaminated, untreated foods, in which they are invariably housed.

Their purpose in the scheme of things is to free the diversified elements in combination, so that they can in turn, form other combinations when they find their way into the intestines, and therefore, ultimately, through the intestinal walls, through the permeable membranes and then into the blood stream itself.

These colloids, elements, food or other things you may call them can then be readily picked up by the body membranes, capillaries, lymph glands, etc., and thus be equitably and properly distributed throughout the body, to maintain, build, repair or regenerate the cells of the organs and tissues as is required by an active, healthy human body.

## CAUSE AND EFFECT

When someone tells me that he or she is unable to eat raw lettuce, or raw cabbage, or any other natural food, I usually ask him to elucidate, and give me a little more data and information, because this vitally interests me. So they usually go on, and tell me the why's and wherefore's and the story usually goes something like this, "Well, if I eat a bit of raw cabbage, boy, do I suffer indigestion — it just about kills me!"

Well, I've sought for an answer to this unusual bodily reaction, and no one seems to know what it's all about; but I don't think it is either that deep or profound or difficult. To me, it just means that the gastro-intestinal bacterial flora that handle the digestive processes of that specific food, are either dead, inert or absent. Well, whether dead, inert or absent, it is caused by one of two things.

1. That you seldom, if ever eat that food, and therefore no bacterial intestinal floral pattern has been established or is available and, therefore, must first be propagated.

2. If you do eat that specific food occasionally, it is because that intestinal bacterial flora is being inhibited, rendered inactive or being killed outright.

Well then, how could this be killed by action of the human body? To begin with, it is not by action of the human body that the flora are killed. I suggest the person may be (a) a heavy drinker of spirituous wines, beers or liquors; (b) a heavy smoker; (c) he may be a fruit farmer who uses a lot of spray, and the inhaling of the spray fumes can do the same trick in a most deadly manner. Then too, this bacterial flora can be killed by some of the heavily chemically treated foods that we put into our stomachs, also the use of hydrogenated oils, mineral oils, drugs, antibiotics, mouth washes, gargles and other germicides and breath purifiers that are very widely used. The means and methods of correction shouldn't be too difficult, if you have good common sense and a little bit of initiative.

The system of putting the sufferer on a diet that avoids these trouble-causing foods is nonsensical and stupid for it only worsens the condition and does not eliminate the cause. I go even further and suggest that these bland, all cooked, chemically treated, nutrition-lacking diets are simply slow death from nutritional starvation.

## ENZYMIC ACTION

Let us not assume that any one enzyme can do a job in itself, because most enzymic action comprises the work of many enzymes. Here I want to cite some examples.

While each kind of enzyme regulates a specific chemical action, as a rule enzymes act in groups or a system . . . and to this date many more than a thousand of these systems have been identified.

Take, for example, the brewing industry. In the process that changes malt and hops to beer, there are fourteen steps or courses and the process of fermentation of sugar to yield alcohol directly involves at least twelve enzymes.

Yes, and while we are giving examples, to break down fats at least nine enzymes are required.

Enzymes are the means of disintegrating the dead and worn out cells, making it possible for the blood to carry them away and excrete them. Other enzymes are responsible for the clotting of blood.

168

When you have an itch, take care. It is caused by enzymes breaking down protein particles in your body. It may and usually does indicate that something is amiss.

The very basis of life — conception — could not take place without enzymic action. Without the part that enzymes play, the male sperm could not pierce and enter the ovum.

It is related that each nerve impulse produces a substance that an enzyme must decompose before another impulse can be transmitted.

It is my firm belief that lack of enzymes in the daily diet contributes to arteriosclerosis, heart disease and other coronary troubles. I believe that the cholesterol build-up in the arteries of the human being is invariably caused by consuming fats without enzymes which the body enzymes cannot break up and they are thus stored or built up in the liver and blood vessels.

This same principle is followed in dealing with hydrogenated fats, for they are similar to plastic and are referred to as plastics in various bulletins, papers and communications. And as plastics, the body enzymes are unable to cope with them. Thus, they are stored or accumulated in the blood vessels where eventually they pile up to such an extent they clog up the artery, a rupture results, followed by clotting . . . and there you have it!

If fats containing enzymes were eaten, as unpasteurized and unhomogenized milk, butter and cheese, the enzymes contained in these foods would properly disseminate the natural fat and make it available for proper distribution throughout the body . . . and thus, make the chemical constituents of fat available to all body organs. The regular use of grains and nuts containing large percentages of unsaturated, natural fats in the diet would be of significant help. If natural food of this kind were used, there would then be no excessive build-up of cholesterol granules in the arteries to cause rupture, clotting and heart attacks.

The matter, to a great deal, rests on the fact that it is not digestion that is important to the human body — but utilization!

In *Consumers Bulletin*, September 1957 issue, an article entitled "The Food You Eat" quotes from statements made by Dr. Tom Douglas Spies at the 1957 Annual Meeting of the American Medical Association as follows:

"All diseases are caused by chemicals, and all diseases can be cured by chemicals. All the chemicals used by the body — except for the oxygen which we breathe and the water which we drink — are taken in through food. If we only knew enough, all diseases could be prevented, and could be cured, through proper nutrition . . .

"As tissues become damaged, they lack the chemicals of good nutrition, they tend to become old. They lack what I call 'tissue integrity'. There are people of forty whose brains and arteries are senile. If we can help the tissues repair themselves by correcting nutritional deficiencies, we can make old age wait."

I suggest that the 'tissue integrity' to which he refers depends upon enzymes as found in natural food.

Co-enzymes are aides to enzymes, related to enzymes, akin to enzymes . . . yet they are not completely enzymes in themselves. Little is known about them but they do work in conjunction with enzymes.

They are described as dialyzable, heat stable organic compounds necessary for the functioning of enzymes. They are associated with, but generally separable from, enzymes. The chemical nature of the enzymic action depends upon the co-enzyme.

I have as yet found no scientific laboratory indication as to whether or not body enzymes are required for the normal assimilation of enzyme-containing food by the body. However I do believe the production of gastric juices and saliva as well as other body functions are performed by synthesized body enzymes. Therefore, I contend that a steady continued intake of enzyme-containing foods is essential for maintenance of the enzyme-synthesizing process.

At this stage, upon making inquiries from those who are supposedly versed in nutrition — even your doctor or your dentist or some other health official — you will be told that the body is capable of synthesizing its own enzymes. However, this is only partially true. The body is capable of synthesizing some enzymes ... but some enzymes are not sufficient to maintain health and well-being. They are not capable of regenerating all the cells and keeping them in perfect order. And the fewer enzymes you take into your body, the less able your body is to synthesize enzymes. Further, as you grow older the body losses its ability to synthesize its own enzymes.

Therefore, when anyone tries to appease you by telling you that the body is capable of synthesizing enzymes, you are being told half a story to lull you into a false sense of security.

Enzymes are nature's handymen. They are the wheels that keep the cycle of life going around. They perform this selfsame duty in the body. They break down the food into components that the body can readily utilize, which means that all of the value contained in the food is placed at the disposal of the body by means of these enzymes.

It is by means of enzymes that the components of food are broken down so that each part, each muscle, each strand and each capillary will receive proper nourishment. Thus the body is able to regenerate itself in perpetuity ... and good health is the result.

Enzymes build muscles. Enzymes store food both in the liver and in the muscles. Enzymes cause the formation of uric acid so that it can be eliminated in the urine. Enzymes help build phosphorus in the bones. Enzymes fix the blood in the red blood cells. It is by means of enzymes that all the body's functions are carried out.

It would take volumes to illustrate all of the functions performed by enzymes.

## RESULTS OF ENZYME DEFICIENCY

Even though many doctors, nutritionists, biochemists, health officials and other supposedly learned people may try to tell you the body can manufacture sufficient enzymes to look after its needs, I want to stand boldly before you and warn you and say, "Do not believe it!"

That the body can make its own enzymes sufficiently to take care of all your body needs is a lie ... and believing and abiding by such can lead you to ill health and untimely death.

Again I want to emphasize that the digestive secretions, fluids and tissues of the animal body are positively not endowed with sufficient enzymes to carry out their functions without aid. Your body requires all the natural enzymes found in proper wholesome, untreated, unmolested food. The enzymes found in natural food are positively and unequivocally not superfluous. They are needed to perform the purpose that nature intended ... and that is why nature put them there.

I would like to quote from the lecture of Dr. Edward Howell, biochemist: "Industrial chemists have discovered the presence of enzymes in a large variety of food materials. But in the meantime investigators in the medical sciences were also busy. I have discovered numerous physicians and laboratory workers reporting the presence of an enzyme deficiency in various body fluids and tissues in human patients and even in apparently healthy human beings. Medical literature, it is true, has been reporting an enzyme deficiency during the past few years, but the defection has been usually mistakenly referred to the pancreas. I maintain, on the basis of much competent evidence, that this deficiency is traceable ultimately to the fact that 'civilized' diet does not contribute the normal quota of enzymes."

As I have related elsewhere in this book, enzymes stand apart from all other food factors in one clear-cut respect. They are invariably extremely sensitive to heat.

Let me further point out that minerals do not lose their identity when they are heated. Neither do vitamins lose their identity, nor are they seriously harmed in the process of cooking. Whether or not they are available or can be assimilated by the body under the circumstances is extremely doubtful. But enzymes are completely destroyed at normal cooking temperatures.

It was a sad day for mankind when primitive man learned to cook his food, for many of the ills and diseases which

172

afflict mankind today are caused by the foods that are consumed by people in America and that are contributors to our ill health would, if they contained their original enzymes, contribute to our well-being.

You can eat any amount of the so called best foods that have been processed, treated or cooked and yet your body will absorb little or none of their nutrient value.

If and when the cause, effect and cure of cancer are discovered, I suspect that the lack of enzymes in food and the body will be of prime or of foremost importance. I further believe that time will prove that most or all cancers could have been prevented or avoided if enzymes had been there to fulfil their proper function.

It is claimed that the reason Eskimos, living in a land where the conditions are the most difficult of all the lands inhabited by human beings and where food is the scarcest and hardest to come by, live in comparative good health to a ripe old age is because a high proportion of their food is eaten raw or comparatively so ... and naturally loaded with enzymes. Blubber, which is a vital part of their diet and is considered a delicacy, is uncooked.

From close observations made of the diet and health of primitive Eskimos, it was revealed that these people eat up to 10 lbs. of raw fish or meat each day. Most nutritionists and physicians contend that such a heavy protein diet will quickly result in high blood pressure, arthritis, kidney trouble and other disorders. I would also like to add that not only are Eskimos comparatively free of all of these diseases in their own environment, but tooth decay is practically unknown among them as well.

Furthermore, when these same Eskimos are transplanted into civilization, the state of their health rapidly deteriorates and most of them get sick or die. This is obviously due to the changeover from their natural, normal diet of chiefly raw or partially cooked foods to the large quantities of cooked and chemically treated foods that they partake of in civilization.

Everyone is acquainted with the longevity and the good health of the Bulgarian peasants and Dr. Edward Howell,

173

the famous biochemist who has done prodigious work in the study of enzymes, states that in his opinion the long life of the Bulgarian peasant is due to the fact that the diet is composed mainly of raw milk, butter and cheese, which not only are high in calories but also contain a proportionate amount of enzymes — because their milk, butter and cheese are not pasteurized and the enzymes are alive and active.

In one most interesting study to illustrate and point out how enzyme-deficiency affects the life span and causes organic diseases, comparisons were made of the pancreas of a sheep with that of a man double the weight of the animal. In this case the pancreas of the sheep weighed 18 grams while that of the human was five times as heavy. The sheep, because it eats grass and only natural living food, got all its natural enzymes with its food and so it made very little demand on the enzymes of the body for digestion ... whereas the man, living on mostly cooked, processed and treated foods, used up and depleted his body enzymes — even with the aid of a huge pancreas which is supposed to be the important part of man's enzyme making machinery.

Another illustration was taken when comparisons were made of the pancreas of Malays who live almost solely on cooked rice as compared with the pancreas of Americans whose diet is somewhat mixed, being cooked and raw. The study illustrated that the pancreas of the Malays was 50% bigger than that of the Americans.

Up until a few years ago zoo keepers throughout the world found great trouble in keeping their animals alive and healthy for any long period. Furthermore, seldom ever did the animals give birth to young in captivity. But since they've learned a little bit about diet and have been giving these animals more and more raw food, conditions have changed. The animals are in much better physical condition and they give birth occasionally to young — alive and healthy.

To illustrate the extreme need and value of enzymes, I again wish to quote from Dr. Edward Howell's bulletin:

"In the past, physicians occasionally used enzymes palliatively to control symptoms. The possibility of an enzyme deficiency in the organism has not been established or even suspected. Now, physicians are justified in employing enzymes as supplemental dietary substances in replacement therapy, parallelled with vitamin therapy. The mass of evidence I have succeeded in assembling places food enzymes in a scientifically ordained category. When a patient with symptoms traceable to the gastrointestinal tract presents himself, every physician should ask the question: Could these symptoms originate from a decrease in the enzymic power of the digestive secretions? Theoretically the answer may be found in actual laboratory examination of the digestive secretions, but in practice this is not feasible. The digestive fluids, particularly the intestinal juice, do not easily lend themselves to accurate evaluation of the enzyme constituents. If it is taken as an assumption that the enzymic efficiency of the gastro-intestinal system tends to be subnormal, it becomes evident that enzyme therapy offers a more scientific approach to the problem than is possible with alkali medication and other palliatives."

At this stage I would like to make a further quotation ... and this is from the magazine *Let's Live*, October 1959 issue, and the heading is "Enzyme lack is leukemia cause":

"Washington, D.C. — One of the major causes of leukemia is an enzyme lack, according to Dr. William Dameshek, of Boston, speaking recently to a professional group.

"He explained that certain agents, such as chemicals, induce deletion of an enzyme which is essential to normal growth of the cell and that in the absence of the enzyme, a new and metabolically different race of cells grows in the form of leukemia."

It has also been phrased that if there are insufficient enzymes taken into the body and the body enzymes are over-taxed, gastrointestinal diseases will result — followed by other ailments.

It is true that through the work of enzymes the natural chemicals or elements in food are made available and assimilable to and by the human system and the body cells, which make up the human body.

It is my belief and conviction, based upon reading, observations, inquiries and studies, that so many people who are tired, listless, worn out, fagged or befuddled are suffering from "enzyme lack".

Because most of their food is processed or cooked, their bodies are devoting their best efforts to synthesizing enzymes. Thus, they have no "steam" left to prepare the essential body forces that are required for normal activity.

One report stated that many researchers are convinced that virtually all disease traces to missing or faulty enzymes.

There has been little or no doubt in my mind for some years that practically all disease known to man is due to the lack of or interference with enzymes.

But don't let anyone try to make you believe that synthetic enzymes are the answer. Remember, each to its own — the natural way.


## AGEING AND ENZYMES

Back in 1912, Casimir Funk, the famed American biochemist, realized the fact that foods contain other substances besides proteins, fats and carbohydrates. He designated these substances by the term vitamins, which he created by combining the word "vite" for life with "amine".

Now you can find these so called vitamins sold and offered in pills, tablets and who knows what other form. It is my belief that this is a gigantic hoax, for in most cases these synthetic vitamins and whatever they might contain are not assimilable or incorporated into the body by the human system. Therefore, the taking of them is a waste of time. I am not sure whether or not they cause injury, but as it is my definite belief that they contribute little or nothing to the health and welfare of the human body, they can only do harm.

Therefore, I suggest that you look with suspicion and doubt upon pills, drugs, synthetics and such, containing supposed vitamins.

176

Vitamins, when found where they belong — in natural foods — are a different story entirely.

Experts on nutrition who have conducted experiments find it is necessary to heat some vitamins at boiling or steam pressure temperatures for many hours before there is complete destruction. Vitamin C is, however, somewhat less resistant to heating than other vitamins ... whereas enzymes, the true, definite and certain life elements, are wholly destroyed by but a few minutes of boiling or cooking.

It is emphasized and accepted that the more enzymes we put into our body, the less stress and strain required by the body to manufacture the enzymes for itself with which to utilize the food that it has taken in.

This can be readily understood and accepted without too much imagination. It is not merely a matter of digestion of food, but utilization which is most important. With the proper intake of enzymes there is no doubt whatsoever about the proper dissemination, distribution and utilization of the food by the body.

There is a school of chemistry that maintains that chemists soon will be able to create or synthesize enzymes in the laboratory. Well, far be it from me to disillusion the chemits and the scientists or to try to minimize their value and importance, but when the time comes that chemists can create living enzymes in the laboratory, then there will be no longer any need for sex, God or a Creator, for the chemist will then fulfil all of these functions.

It is my contention that deficiency of enzymes in the body, which eventually spells the inability of the body to synthesize proper sufficient enzymes, is the prime cause of early ageing, or to put it simply, getting old before your time.

Premature cellular exhaustion is said to be the cause of many of the troubles of the human race, and this condition is brought about by the lack of enzymes in the food that is consumed. Thus the necessity of the body to work overtime and over-exert itself to make these required enzymes.

It is clearly and definitely established that as we grow

older, the body gradually loses its ability to synthesize enzymes. Scientists at the world famous Michael Reese Hospital in Chicago found that old people had less than 1/30th as many enzymes in the saliva as young people.

Then, too, Dr. Eckardt of Germany discovered, after 1200 tests, that enzymes found in the urine were only half the number in old people as in young people. I stress that it can be readily understood how essential it is for one's health to maintain the continued intake of enzymes in your food ... and the need grows more pressing with age.

Further, Dr. Burge of the University of Illinois found, upon doing some work with potato beetles, that the old potato beetles had less than half as many enzymes as the younger fellows.

Dr. Sekla, Charles University, Prague found the same thing true when he worked with fruit flies. Then Dr. Falk and his associates did another experiment of a similar nature on rats. In both of these species the enzymes began to weaken after middle age.

Here let me press home a warning. Don't wait to start getting more enzymes when you are older, for by then you may have lost your teeth and you will be unable to readily and properly masticate the food that contains sufficient enzymes.

In a discussion some time ago with one who was well versed in nutrition, he said that youth and old age can be summed up in this way, "When you are young, you put more enzymes into your body's bank of enzymes, and as you grow older, the tendency is to eat more cooked foods and there you are drawing on body enzymes. When the time comes that you are drawing out more than you are putting in, that is the positive indication that old age is creeping up on you."

Therefore, it follows that death is the result when you have overdrawn your enzyme bank account and the various organs cannot be maintained. Thus, they fail to function and then comes the end. So it can be clearly seen that enzymes are the key to life.

Now as we have clearly illustrated, enzymes do most of

the work of metabolizing and digesting, which means simply that the proper chemical changes are being made from food to living cells.

Here is a most interesting development.

It has not been proven that enzymes are used up, for, as it is related, enzymes are supposed to act only as a catalyst — without themselves being used up in the process. However, it is a fact that when the food is excreted, the enzymes go along with the remains of the food. This includes the body enzymes that were synthesized and used in digesting the food.

Now if this is maintained over a long period of time, exhaustion of body enzymes will eventually occur. Thus, as you grow older, your quota of body enzymes becomes smaller and eventually death takes over. Thus, it cannot be denied that you are as old as your enzymes.

It can be understood that where there are not enough enzymes in the stomach and bowels to properly digest your food, enzymes will be drawn from other parts of the body — such as glands, muscles, nerves and even from the blood. This clearly indicates that eventually there will be a deficiency of enzymes in these organs and other functional body structures and a broad variety of ailments usually follows.

Thus, I stress the importance of maintaining the supply of natural enzymes along with your food if you wish to extend your life span and remain free of disease and be in good health.

No one can deny that nature intended that a human being remain in good health ... and this can be done by the simple expedient of making sure that the foods that you put into your body contain living enzymes as provided by nature.

Lack of or presence of enzymes is the true reason why some men are old at forty and others are young at seventy-five.

When it is realized that most of our modern foods are void of enzymes, it can then be accepted that synthesized enzymes are constantly being used up every day and voided in the urine and the stool. Thus, the possibility that the enzyme potential may be strained past the danger point can be understood and accepted.

By maintaining a regular diet consisting chiefly of enzyme-containing natural foods, you can defeat or hold off old age. The solution is, I believe, a simple one. Maintain a heavy intake of natural foods containing enzymes and you can hold old age at bay — beyond the promised three score and ten.

Now we run into a sort of analogy.

With those of us who consume large quantities of enzymeless foods, like cooked, processed and treated foods, as compared to someone whose intake of food in general is light, here we see now why slender people or people of light weight seem to be healthier and live longer than people who are big and thus consume much more food. The man with the large food consumption uses up more of his body enzymes and thus, when these enzymes are depleted, disease and death are the result.

The greater the amount of food consumed, especially the cooked foods, the greater the amount of enzymes that must be produced by the body and wasted in the process of excretion.

Experiments on insects have indicated that when the body enzymes are used at a rapid rate, there is an earlier onset of old age and death. There is indicated in the same research the possibility of increasing the span of life to new horizons by exploring and experimenting more deeply in the study of enzymology . . . and the researcher who devotes his time to this may reach great fame and renown.

When you adopt a diet of cooked foods or foods that contain little or no enzymes, you are forcing yourself into a positive starvation regimen that can result in but one thing . . . ill health and untimely death.

We know from the old story of life that as we grow older we tend to get grey, our hair falls out, we get wrinkles, we get stiff in the joints, our muscles sag, our eyes lose their capacity to see clearly and the brightness disappears. We look played out, bedraggled and we have lost our pep and our zest for living. It is my humble opinion that this process is due to the lack or shortage of enzymes in the body.

It appears reasonable, from my survey and study of the situation, that the sure, the certain and the safe way to maintain your health and hold off old age is to eat foods rich in enzymes — foods that will contribute to the welfare and well-being of one's body. The answer is uncooked foods, natural foods — foods that have not been treated or heated in any manner, shape or form.

# CHAPTER 13

## Deadly Margarine and Fats

*"It is advisable not only to avoid any visible solid fats but to
eliminate them in our cooking by not eating foods fried in saturated
fats. Broil foods, so that if there is any fat in them it will melt off."*

....: DR. MORRIS BRAND

### GUARD YOUR OWN

Just a few days ago a good friend of mine jokingly said,
"Well, Friend Tobe, I know you'll like me ... I use
nothing but pure 100% corn oil margarine."

"Well," I replied, "that's as good a way to kill yourself
as any way I know. You'll get a heart attack quicker from
it than you will from good wholesome farmer's butter."

My friend looked at me in utter amazement. "Why, I
thought you told me that animal fats caused heart attacks
and arteriosclerosis and such."

"Yes," I replied, "I am guilty of making that statement ... and I still believe that an over-abundance of the
animal fats, the saturated type, will cause heart disease."

My friend hurriedly put in, "So now where am I?
Here I am using pure corn oil margarine and you say that
it's no good or worse than the other."

With a dejected sigh, I said, "Circumstances don't
allow me to go into any great detail but here's something
for you to think about ... If that margarine is pure corn
oil, or any other vegetable oil, how come you buy it in
that nice solid brick form, so to speak? What kind of
mumbo-jumbo or mystic wand waving turns the fluid oil
into a solid mass?"

"Mmm, hmmm," replied my friend. "That's a good
question."

It's not the pure corn oil that I'm objecting to ... it's
the treatment to which it's subjected, and the process
referred to as hydrogenation. And I want to tell you
this ... *that's* the killer diller, the dastardly dirk, the

182

bogey man . . . and Nick Carter, Sherlock Holmes, Ellery Queen and Perry Mason all snooping together couldn't lay him by the heels either.

Lest you think I'm barking up the wrong tree or don't know my petunias from onions, go to the library and get a book on food processing or write to the Department of Health and ask them to explain to you in detail what the process of hydrogenation consists of. When you've done this and given the matter some study, if you still want to eat margarine or any other food containing hydrogenated oil (and there are many, many such foods) then that's your privilege. But brother, you're going to be dead a lot quicker than if you'd let them alone.

Better still, ask for and get a sample of hydrogenated peanut or other vegetable or animal oil, and examine it with your own eyes and hands.

Here is my concocted definition of the process of hydrogenation. And I warn you that this is not necessarily the scientific or dictionary explanation of the meaning of hydrogenation . . . it's just what I say it is.

"The Process of Hydrogenation . . . converts a natural animal or vegetable oil into a synthetic fat or plastic. I further contend that this synthetic fat or plastic, when consumed or taken into the body, raises the blood cholesterol level — apart from any other harm it may inflict upon the body."

Then my friend put in, with a serious look on his face, "Why aren't we told about this?"

And I countered, "You tell me! Whose duty do you think it is to tell you about these things?"

"Then why doesn't the government do something about protecting us?"

"Maybe the government doesn't think that it's harmful."

"But is it harmful?" my friend pressed.

"In my humble opinion, it is not only positively harmful, but devastating."

So my friend left me, scratching his head and wondering and my parting remark was this, "If you don't make it a point to find out, if you don't search and study and learn, then you deserve the untimely death that you're going to meet ... and don't look for the government or anyone else to protect you."

## MAKING OILS SOLID

It is suggested that the reason the hydrogenation process is so widely used in the food industry is that it makes all oils look, act and taste alike.

Therefore, whether the original oil is fresh, stale, rancid, old, dirty, discolored — peanut, corn, sunflower, olive, beef, swine or sheep — when the process of hydrogenation is through with it, along with its kindred processing like preserving, filtering, denaturing, deodorizing and bleaching, 'tis as white and crystal-like as the newly fallen snow.

You see, hydrogenated oil is useless as far as food is concerned, and what is even worse — harmful — for it is nothing but a plastic. And top-ranking authorities today claim that it is one of the potent causes of arteriosclerosis and heart attacks.

If the human system can digest and assimilate hydrogenated oils or foods treated by the hydrogenation process then it should or would be capable of digesting and assimilating the other plastics used in industry.

Now, hydrogenated oils are widely used in many of your foods. Our government and the food rules and regulations do not demand that it be stated on the package if hydrogenated oil is used. However, to the best of my knowledge and belief, no oil like shortening and margarine can be made to stand up in the package unless it is hydrogenated. It is the process of hydrogenation that allows the miracle to happen — that is, the melting point is increased so that a flowing oil will stand up and it becomes semi-solid or solid.

Hydrogenated oil as a food is in clear-cut simple language, an unmitigated counterfeit.

# ARE ANIMAL FATS O.K.?

One of the greatest evils in our diet, if not the greatest of all, is the use of animal fat of any kind . . . that is, the fat derived from the carcass of any animal. This, I am sorry to admit, must include butter. It would not include milk but it would include cream. You see, milk is the whole product as excreted by the mammary glands of the animal, whereas cream is a fragmented food. I urge you to shun all fragmented foods. Cream and butter or cheese are fragmented foods and by that I mean incomplete, and therefore do not deserve a place in the diet of human beings or animals.

I stoutly contend that if it were not for the use of animal fats such as cream, butter, cheese, fat meat and eggs, as well as margarine, there would be little danger of any human being ever having a heart attack. I place margarine in the same class as an animal fat because it has been chemically hardened or saturated. In fact, I consider it by far the worst of all fats. Yes, diseases of the heart would cease to be a threat against the very existence of mankind if these fats were shunned.

Thus, I join in this chorus and say to you, "If you will attain health and long life, you must immediately forego the use of any form of animal fats." And I say this in spite of the advice of famous nutritionists and your various government health agencies who tell you to use eggs, cream, butter and cheese . . . as well as margarine. Milk is the least harmful but it definitely is not a good or health-giving food.

I suggest that you make your own studies and observations, and your conclusions cannot differ too much from mine.

# CHAPTER 14

## Mental Health

> *"Nutrition directly affects growth, development, reproduction, well-being and the physical and mental condition of the individual. Health depends upon nutrition more than on any other single factor."*
>
> ; ; ; . DR. WM. H. SEBRALL, JR.

## MENTAL AND EMOTIONAL ASPECTS OF HEALTH

Here we are dealing with one of the most complicated and difficult aspects of health.

The study and practice of psychology has grown tremendously in the past two or three decades, which leads one to believe that there are more emotional or mental upsets among the populace than in previous times... which is probably true. The reasons for the increase in the number of people with mental problems are given as "stress" and "the rat race" and "the pressures of modern-day living".

Now here at the start I want to emphasize that it is my sincere belief that most mental ailments are basically physical. I contend it is difficult, if not impossible, to find a deranged mind and a healthy body or vice versa, a sick body and healthy mind ... unless the damage was caused by accident, prenatally or at birth. There are many mental conditions that are caused in this manner.

However, my investigations would suggest that in most cases the problem is physical and when the body has been brought back to good health, the mental situation clears up on its own.

I fully realize that when dealing with human emotions such as jealousy, hate, desire, love, anger and passion, the physical aspect would appear to have little or no value or meaning. I do suggest, however, that if a body is in good physical condition, properly nourished and rested, when an emotional problem arises the human being so fortified is in a better position to withstand the shock or face up to the problem at hand. Thus, with rational thinking, any serious consequences can generally be prevented.

I reiterate this as being my experience, after watching and noting and observing for most of my lifetime.

You may say, and justifiably, that when one is upset emotionally he cannot eat properly or rest properly and therefore the entire structure is thrown out of balance — which, in turn, aggravates the mental condition. Now please follow me and I will try to explain what I mean.

Here I'd like to cite as an example a story which is basically true and which may throw some light on the subject. I have been in active business for almost forty years ... that is, since the days of my youth ... and I have faced and encountered many, many frustrating emotional situations, circumstances and problems. They run the gamut of practically all of the emotions common to normal man but most of my problems evolved around finances and love. Perhaps that strikes a respondent chord in the minds of most of my readers.

Based on my experiences and reading, I contend forcibly that invariably sound, sane thinking will correct the trouble. But, you might ask, at certain times who is capable of sane, sound thinking and reasoning. And I reply, if you are properly nourished and rested, you will be in a position to master the problems that face you. It may be difficult, it may be trying, but you will surmount them.

At one time, like 90% or more of all the people in America, I too enjoyed my weekends. It is a fact, and I'm sure you will recognize it, that most of the fun and the drinking and the smoking and the sex and the over-eating take place on weekends. And I am sure you know that most younger people (and many not so young) can hardly wait for Friday night to arrive so they can begin their over-indulgences.

During the summer many or most of these excesses take place at the summer cottage, away from the eyes of close friends, relatives and business associates. Well, under such a pattern of living — you know, with the whooping it up that goes on Friday night, Saturday day and night and Sunday — well, on Monday morning one isn't usually at the peak of efficiency, either mentally or physically. There's no doubt about it, that is where "blue Monday" had its origin.

From many years' experience as an employer I have found that there is less work done Monday morning than any other day of the week, except perhaps late Friday afternoon when everybody is anxious to get away to start the cycle over again . . . and they fidget and put in their time with bated breath till the hour of their emancipation arrives.

There is a school of thought that is quite prevalent in America that maintains that stress and strain and our present-day way of life are the cause of heart disease and other illnesses.

If the good doctor or researcher or whoever it may be who is building up this theory on the mental stress aspect is seeking to blame our over-indulgences like liquor, smoking, coffee and other contaminated foods, then I would go along with him and agree with him whole-heartedly. Frankly, I think that is what the doctor means without saying so.

He does not want to point his finger directly at these conditions for fear of involving himself in a battle with the powerful multi-million dollar corporations. After all, researchers are most reluctant to bite the hand that feeds them . . . for no one can deny that the fertilizer, the drug, the processed food and the chemical food industries are the greatest contributors to the welfare and prosperity of the healing and research groups like universities and such. It ill behooves these gentlemen to point an accusing finger at them. Anyone with an ounce of normal grey matter can see the truth of my assertion.

So instead, they blame the stress and strain and the hazards and pressures of modern day living. They don't go out on a limb and say specifically that it is the products produced by these powerful moneyed manufacturing interests that are the cause of the disorders.

It is my positive conviction that stress is not a factor where other conditions of proper living are satisfactory. I have known cases where bad news, the report of a death of a loved one or a deteriorating financial condition has brought about the onset of certain diseases. As a matter of fact, I have witnessed such situations as they were actually created. But it is my contention that in every case where this occurred the person involved was already suffering from or already in the throes of an advanced condition of this disease and it was only the shock that brought it to light or necessitated the attendance of a doctor who found the condition. I maintain the condition was there for some time prior to shock. The shock just made it evident.

Worry has long been regarded as one of the curses of civilization which brought deterioration and disarrangement to people's minds. I cannot agree with this thesis. To me, worry means facing problems of varying seriousness and finding a means and a way of coping with them. The worry of today brings the solution of tomorrow.

I am not talking about the so-called worrywart who worries about tomorrow's weather or whether the Yankees will win the World Series or whether war will break out or whether his children will be called up for active service and eventually be wounded or killed. With such cases I am not concerned. They are trivial and specifically of one's own making and do not deserve the consideration or the understanding of normal, sensible individuals. If people have nothing else to worry about then I would humbly suggest that they occupy themselves with more important considerations involving life and living.

I know, too, that sexual problems confront millions of American men and women . . . and here again, the food pattern and the way of living are both the cause and the solution.

It must not be ignored that the excessive use or even the continued use of tobacco, drugs, alcohol and coffee will positively cause mental and emotional disorders. Investigations will reveal that in most, if not in all cases of mental and emotional upsets one or all of these are involved. The widespread use of synthetic drugs probably heads the list as the source of these derangements. I would rank the drugs far above alcohol.

It is an absolute fact that we all suffer to a greater or lesser degree from our emotions. The sight of someone being injured or killed, the news of catastrophe and such happenings have different effects upon different individuals.

I have watched the behaviour of a family — a large family of nine children — at the death of a parent. Some wept and moaned and were almost hysterical and carried on with rather violent reactions. Some of the others comforted them and others wept silently and others did not weep at all. It all depends on the degree of control and also on the physical condition of the individual.

For example, at the death of my mother who was 86 years old I felt only the twinge of her parting — of her being taken from us. I saw no reason to shed tears — she had lived her allotted three score and ten, and sixteen extra, and she had been in comparatively good health. My reaction was, "I hope I do as well." But the affection for my mother and the tenderness that I felt towards her still linger in my heart . . . and will remain there until I go to meet her again.

I believe there is also a strong control or binding effect in one's own reasoning mechanism. Tell yourself, "I'm going to hold on to myself. I'm not going to let myself break down and weep and moan. It's stupid — it's nonsensical — it isn't like a rational civilized human being to do that. I'm supposed to be a civilized, knowledgeable human so I must be sure to act like one."

With such reasoning, greater degrees of control can be expected. And I urge my readers to try this means or method when an emotional, upsetting situation arises.

The term "nerves" has been grossly misused and overexaggerated. Practically every condition that human beings suffer, everything they do that shouldn't be done or every action that they perform that is frowned upon is blamed upon nerves. I contend that nerves are nothing else but a degeneration of all body functions and proper food and rest will quickly help correct the situation. The expression "nerves" is an excuse — and a poor one — and to me definitely not acceptable.

I do not suggest that we should try to suppress our emotions. What I am advising is rationalizing with them. If something aggravates me or annoys me, I express myself on the point — sometimes rather vehemently — even in the presence of outsiders. And I make no apologies for it either. Stifling emotions is probably one of the worst things that one can do. But rationalizing them is strictly another matter. I just do not want to go overboard over them and that is where rationalizing is of great help.

It cannot be denied that the emotional aspects have tremendous import and do play a vital part in maintaining the health of a human being. Dr. W. B. Cannon, who did some exceptional experiments at Harvard University clearly revealed the fact that the feelings of love consciously cultivated have the effect of brightening the eyes, improving the circulation, as well as the digestion, and promoting a harmonious functioning of the eliminative system. His research also brought to light the fact that emotions of fear, envy and hate seriously affect the entire body in an exactly opposite manner.

Some scientists would have us believe, and offer rather imposing proof from experiments, that mental upsets can cause many diseases, including stomach ulcers, asthma, skin disorders and heart trouble. Yes, I would agree... but in most cases this is due to a weakened constitution brought about by improper diet and lack of proper sleep and rest.

A well established, supposed authority on mental healing made this statement: "Control of sickness is mental, because sickness itself is mental."

He goes on to state further, "The body of itself has no power to generate disease; it is merely the shadow thrown by mind, and a healthy mind will shadow forth a healthy body."

I most emphatically disagree with this authority. I

191

maintain that the body of itself does have the power to generate disease and all disease is caused from within the body. Therefore, the body creates disease of both physical and mental nature. I further contend that subsequent research, studies and investigations will reveal that my thesis is correct.

There is a school of thought that believes the mind has the power to heal the body and that all disease can be cured and controlled by the mind. I have taken a bit of trouble to investigate this method and means of healing and I find that the writer, in most cases, assumed or considered the body and the mind one and the same thing ... but that the mind is the control system. Well, this is so much like splitting hairs. It has long been my contention that the body controls all the actions and reactions and as the mind is part of the body, then they're one and the same thing.

However, it must be recognized that neither the body nor the mind have the means or the method or the capabilities of creating an element. If calcium or phosphorus or molybdenum or borax is required by the body, the mind or the body itself has no means or method of creating them or synthesizing them. Therefore, they must be brought into the body through natural foods. And if that is done, then of course the body or mind has the ability to retain, regain or maintain health.

Nerves are a part of the body just as muscles, skin, blood, heart, liver and other organs are. They cannot be set apart as though they were an entity apart from the body. Therefore, the things that affect the body affect the nerves. Thus, feed and rest the body, adopt the principles of wholesome natural living, and your nerves will be in sound healthy untroubled condition.

To add weight to my contention that there is no such thing as stress to a properly nourished, well rested and clean living body following the natural living system, I would like to refer you to an experiment conducted by Dr. Agnes Faye Morgan. Her experiments with rats that were found to have damaged glands and the graphic change that took place speak for themselves. When the source of trouble was corrected, that is, by means of supplying the necessary nutrients, the glands, though revealing previous damage, showed that they had been repaired by proper food.

I maintain that we can combat and beat off disease by strengthening the body's own defences against stress. A properly nourished body in a wholesome environment and with proper rest can shake off stress like a duck shakes off water.

## INNOCENT CONDEMNED

I was shocked to learn that in America there are between 5½ to 6 million retarded children. My prayer is, "O Lord, help these children." My more fervent prayer is, "O Lord, prevent this from happening to many more."

Those 5½ to 6 million children are living proof that almost 12,000,000 parents didn't bother to inform themselves concerning health and the proper way of living. These children were not inflicted upon the parents by an act of a vicious creator.

I tell you this, ladies and gentlemen, that the birth of retarded children can be prevented ... and it is oh, so simple. If the parents inform themselves about health, proper nutrition and the proper way of life and then abide by it their children cannot be anything else but healthy. And if they will feed those children on proper food, they will grow up to be healthy.

Please, parents and would-be parents, believe me. Put it to a test. Seek knowledge ... but not the knowledge that you will get from the chemical corporations and the bakery foundations or the food processors or even the governements. Get knowledge that is unshackled, that is untained, that has not been bought and paid for. Get knowledge that is written and prepared by free men who have nothing to gain except to help you gain knowledge.

Any man, any group, any organization that advocates the use of any food that contains chemicals, of any food that is cooked, of any food that contains a preservative is not speaking the truth and he is not advising you in your best interests.

Please, women, would-be mothers, if you are pregnant, don't smoke, don't drink, don't take pills of any kind — I repeat, any kind. They can do naught but harm. I'm not so much concerned about you as individuals — I'm concerned about the unborn children. Give them a fighting chance in life!

# CHAPTER 15

## Sexual Virility

*"Grant me but health, thou great Bestower of it, and give me this fair goddess as my companion."*

. . . . . STERNE

### SEX AND AGE

I must confess that I am no expert when it comes to matters pertaining to sex.

However, I acknowledge that there are many good writers on sex. When I was a young man Havelock Ellis was the authority on eugenics and such. I have read Havelock Ellis, Dr. Herman H. Ruben, Rennie McAndrew, Dr. E. Courtney Beale, E. Parkinson Smith, Anthony Havil, Dr. S. A. Lewin, John Gilmore, Ph.D., Dr. Joseph H. Green, Elliot E. Philipp, M.A., M.D., B.Chir., F.R.C.S., M.R.C.O.G., and others, and they didn't teach me very much that I haven't known for at least forty years. I most certainly do not accept, as do many people, the teachings in the supposedly great volume, "The Kama Sutra", by the great Indian sage, Vatsyayana. It is supposed to be a text book of love and an encyclopedia of sex. I suggest it is grossly over-rated.

I really wonder if anyone knows to any degree of accuracy just how long a man's sexual potency is supposed to last. I have heard various figures suggested. Most people seem to have the idea that a man when he reaches fifty is definitely on the down-grade. Some are a little more generous and will give a man till sixty before he starts to hit the skids.

But I refuse to accept such a verdict. I am judging by the behaviour of animals that I have observed in my lifetime. I have known of tomcats that have been able to perform their sexual functions extremely well until they neared the end of their lives. From my reading of the sexual ways and extension of time of other animals I gather the same impression. Usually the male of the species can perform the sex act until his days on earth are almost finished and I stoutly maintain that this should hold true for human beings as well.

If it doesn't hold true it is because we have abused our bodies. I contend further, that the greatest abuse of our bodies occurs through the medium of incorrect eating or even incorrect drinking — or a combination of both. Remember, no animal on earth drinks or smokes or partakes of chemicals in its food or other contaminatives. Of course, the part about chemicals would not hold true in the case of domesticated animals.

You have all heard the much-used expression that a man is as old as his arteries. Well, I think in the true light of a man's anatomy it should be said that a man is as old as his sex organs and glands.

Isn't it a strange thing that in our society as a man reaches his fourth or fifth and especially his sixth decade, it seems to be expected of him that his sexual interests would decline? If a man of say, 50 or 60 shows interest in a trim ankle or an attractive figure, eyebrows become arched, he is looked down upon, ridiculed or spoken about in a rather insinuative manner. Often one will hear the expression, "There is no fool like an old fool" ... suggesting that sex and sex interests and the thrills found in charm, form and beauty belong to youth and must be denied to anyone who has reached middle age or beyond. I, for one, refuse to accept this restriction. A man of fifty or sixty or even beyond has as much right to be interested in sex as a youth.

To me, sexual drive, like good health, is not just a matter of age. Now I won't go on record as saying that age has nothing whatsoever to do with the situation but I would, in all sincerity, maintain that age has very little to do with sexual prowess.

Because of the controversial aspects of this statement I want to emphasize that I am not talking poppy-cock nor am I referring to something about which I have read. I am actually speaking from experience, from observation, from scientific research data and besides all this I am dealing

196

with facts related to me in intimate conversations and inquiry. It is my belief that the sexual organs, more than any other organ in the human body, are a reflection of the health of the body as a whole.

You see, you may be sick yet your eyesight may be such that you can spot a needle in a haystack. You may be sick and yet your hearing may be so sharp that you can hear a pin drop. You may be sick and still be able to put in a hard day's work. You may be sick and still be able to run, or you may be sick and still be able to eat like a horse. But if you are sick it will be reflected first in your sexual endeavours.

No one can deny that sex plays a more important role in the lives of humanity than any other single factor. Oh yes, I fully realize that there are many men and women among us who have little or no desire for sex. In fact, some, well they just couldn't care less if they ever indulged in sexual congress. Yes, I'd go further and say there are many who prefer definitely not to indulge and may even regard sex as repugnant. Well now, let's be rational and face the truth about these things. If sex is repugnant, there is something radically wrong with the individual whether male or female. Nature provided the sex motivation and made it the strongest of all instincts in the animal kingdom because it was essential for the perpetuation of life.

I have heard it said, and no doubt so have you, for it is a common expression, "If you don't enjoy sexual relations, you are either void of human feeling, a pervert, a homosexual or a lesbian."

Now a good question arises. "Can sexual prowess be retained into ripe old age?" Well, this I can tell you with absolute authority because it turned up in my investigations. I have known both men and women who were still sexually potent in their 80's. I cannot go beyond that age because I haven't had the privilege of talking to people in their 90's and asking these questions. But let me assure you that I have known both men and women who were sexually capable in their 80's.

Now let it be clearly understood that sex was not the

prime motivating factor in their existence at that age but they occasionally still felt the urge and still enjoyed it. It is an absolute fact that there are men of thirty who indulge in sex only occasionally while there are men in their 60's who indulge regularly — every day or every other day. This is not an exaggeration nor an isolated example.

There is a fairly high proportion of men in this world of ours who say that if they no longer can appreciate a trim ankle or a shapely figure or feel an upsurge in their blood-stream when they see an attractive woman, then it would be better for them if life would come to an end. As for me, I don't think that I would say I'd rather be dead if I had no sexual drive or interests but I certainly believe life would lose most of its appeal, most of its pleasure, most of its beauty and yes, fascination.

It is widely accepted that as we grow older our sexual desire or potency diminishes but it is the rate of decline that is the criterion. With most of us the sexual incidence or sexual curve rises sharply from youth into young manhood and then, from what I gather, it remains at the apex for a short period and then declines. When you get to be around forty the decline starts to become quite marked. It is my firm belief that this should not necessarily be true and I am convinced that a man can retain his sexual vigor over a long period of years and I would be so brash as to say that a man's sexual potency should last from about thirteen until at least the age of seventy-five.

The question often arises with men in their 50's or 60's, "Is it possible to overdo sex after one's fifth or sixth decade?" The only positive indication of a vigorous sexual expenditure that I could discover was loss of hair . . . for it is accepted that sexual prowess and baldness go hand in hand. It is my belief that when a man is in normal health and getting proper food and rest, the frequency of sexual orgasms cannot possibly do him any harm whether he enjoys it once a week or every day. If his mind and body feel in the mood I think it is absolutely safe.

It must be remembered that the strongest muscles are those that are used continuously and regularly and the

198

weakest muscles are those that are not used but are neglected and allowed to become decrepit. Therefore, I strongly urge that if you are in the mood and your body and mind call for sex that you indulge with the full knowledge that you are doing the right thing. However, if it interferes with your religious scruples, then that is another story. I suggest that you act as your conscience dictates.

## SEX AND VEGETARIANISM

I have had a fairly wide and yet intimate association with vegetarians. Invariably, it is accepted that because of their vegetarian way of life their sexual incidence and their sexual drive are less than those of men who are meat eaters. In fact, most of the vegetarians of my acquaintance have admitted it and taken it for granted. Many have even offered reasons and justification for this existing condition.

They will say, "Oh, the meats, the fats and the animal products excite the passions but our food is of a different quality, as nature intended and does not create such manifestation."

Well, let me say this. I do not accept this cock-and-bull story . . . from either side of the fence. There is no reason on earth why a vegetarian should not be as virile as any meat eater. In fact, I will stoutly defend a vegetarian against all comers when it comes to sexual or physical prowess. A vegetarian on a proper diet — and I stress proper diet — should be able to out-perform and outlast any normal flesh eater, as he does in all other tests of physical endurance.

Then you may ask, "If what you say is true, then why doesn't it happen? Why don't the vegetarians stand up and defend themselves on these issues?"

My answer to this is that most vegetarians are uninformed concerning what to eat and what will give them proper strength and virility. The average vegetarian cares little and knows little about what he eats — as long as it is not an animal product.

To illustrate how badly the scales are tipped against the

vegetarian, an omnivore can, by just going along the path and following the recommendations of the so-called nutrition experts and the run of the mill diet books, maintain a fair degree of health and virility. But with the vegetarian the situation is entirely different. Because he does not have meat or animal products of any kind he just cannot go along and eat anything at all and expect to be healthy and virile. He must know what he is eating, he must have proper, wholesome food.

This I will tell you and it is as true and sure as the sun rises and sets in the heavens ... a vegetarian whose diet consists chiefly of vegetables that have been cooked, or canned or treated, has about as much chance of having a proper diet as you have of swimming the Atlantic. I repeat, he doesn't have a glimmer of a chance on a cooked food diet!

But, take this selfsame vegetarian and put him on a diet of raw vegetables, raw grains, raw nuts and raw fruits and he'll outrun, outwalk, outwork, outlast and outsex any meat eater on the face of the earth. To verify my statements consult a food chart showing comparative nutrient values of cooked and raw foods. Go down the list and pick out any food you like. Then run across the line and see what it says about the value of this food, cooked and raw, and note the values that are lost in the cooking or treating. That will tell the story.

But there still remains one clincher. Take, for example, apples where it gives you the values raw and cooked. You will see that the cooked apples have practically one half the value of the raw apples. Even though the mineral values are reduced to half for the cooked apple, I want to remind you that this does not give you the whole picture. I maintain that not only has the mineral value been reduced but the reduced portion cannot be properly assimilated by the body. The amount that the body can assimilate from a cooked food is unknown.

I don't know whether or not you understand me in this, so I want to go over it again to make sure that you do understand. Let us say the amount of calcium contained in a fresh raw apricot is 73 units and the amount contained in a cooked apricot is 45. That does not mean that the cooked apricot lis ⅔ as good as the raw apricot . . . no sir by no means! It means that the 73 parts contained in the raw apricot are assimilable by the body but the 45 parts left in the cooked apricot are not necessarily assimilable Perhaps the body can only get 1% or 5% or 20% of that 45. This may sound complicated, but it really isn't. My aim is to indicate in unmistakable parlance the importance of knowledge concerning the value of correct food. The body needs the vital components so readily available in raw foods, and so elusive in cooked foods, to carry on all of its normal functions — including the sex act.

This proves my contention that if you want to be sexually virile or healthy all-round, the way to accomplish this feat is by means of a proper diet and a proper diet means a diet that consists mainly of raw fresh foods in their prime condition.

If you have studied or will study the various matters and principles concerning the heart, heart diseases and cholesterol and such, you will come across this little fact that cholesterol is essential for the sexual well-being of any normal male. It is also a fact that a diet heavy in animal fats — fat meat, butter, milk, cream, cheese and eggs — creates a surplus of cholesterol in the human body. Therefore, it might be assumed or expected that if cholesterol contributes to the sex drive, meat eaters who eat all these foods we mentioned will have a greater sex drive than those who don't. This bit of vital information is made capital of by those who would justify flesh eating or attempt to prove its superiority over the vegetarian way of life.

But there is a fallacy here which I would like to bring to your attention. First, let me point out that if you do have a diet heavy in animal fats the chances are you won't be able to live beyond 50 or 60 because you are a prime candidate for heart attack. So therefore, if you are seeking to improve your sexual position, you may wind up shortening it drastically by means of a heart attack — a thrombosis or a coronary. However, an investigation into body chemistry will quickly reveal that the human body is capable ot making all the cholesterol that is required for the body's needs without one fragment of animal fat being added to the body in the form of food. Now this again is an absolute scientific principle and can be verified by digging into various research experiments.

## SEX AND HUNGER

Just how does hunger affect a man's sexual activity? Can a man who is starved sustain a regular sexual output?

One would imagine that a person who is properly nourished would have a higher sexual average than a person who was hungry or starved. Actual statistics and clinical research have little to offer on this subject. One authority claims that food hunger actually is anti-aphrodisiacal and this theory has substantial backing from authorities on fasting. Anyone who has undergone a fast will attest to the fact that while undergoing the fast, sexual libido drops to a low, low ebb. On the other hand, it is a known fact that in both China and India where lack of food and starvation are generally accepted, the number of births is far above that in the countries where food is plentiful. For example, you can compare this to the Nordic lands or to Canada, Australia and New Zealand where there is no shortage of food and the birth rate is low. So there is a bit of room for conjecture or argument. Furthermore, it is another generally known fact that the most sexually vigorous men are the slender men.

It has been my experience in dealing with seeds and plants and trees — in fact, throughout my whole study of botany — that plants that are undernourished or growing under adverse conditions will, in many cases, set seed sooner and more prodigiously than a well nourished plant grown in more fertile ground.

Who can deny that among humans the sex instinct is much stronger than it is among animals? Again, here conclusive proof is difficult to obtain. But we do know that man is capable of indulging around the calendar which no animal can do. The reason given for the belief that the sex instinct is much stronger in man is based upon the fact that a human being has a most vivid imagination, which is a faculty that animals do not possess. Imagination and mental stimulus can be a potent factor in arousing the sex desire to fever pitch. Furthermore, man of all the creatures on earth has learned to derive a great deal of pleasure from the sex act and accepts it as a prime source of delight. But man goes far beyond that, for he also incorporates with it such divine manifestations as love, tenderness, sympathy, yearning, romance, devotion and all that is beautiful and noble in life. So this must be regarded as evidence that the sex urge of the human being is many, many times greater than that found in animals.

Is it not true that the sex act taken seriously by both man and woman can, by intelligent manipulation, become a most heavenly and pleasurable experience? This is especially so where both parties lend themselves thoroughly to the play and the act. Who can deny that when a man and a woman are deeply in love with each other and joined together in sexual union, they have reached the loftiest pinnacle which human beings can attain? It is then and then only that man and woman merge into one.

It is generally accepted that in infancy and early childhood food is the most important thing in life. Then around the age of puberty and perhaps into manhood, sex seems to become more important than food. After one reaches perhaps the fourth or fifth decade of life, sex becomes less important and food once more emerges as the greater force. This, too, is of course debatable because I have known men in their sixth and seventh decades of life who did not consider food of very great importance. I submit, however, that only when the sex urge has vanished does the pleasure of eating assume an important role.

## IMPOTENCY AND STERILITY

Nowhere is it established or known just what comprises

a man's normal sexual frequency. Nowhere can I find anything that even resembles an established figure.

Martin Luther considered once a month the proper number, whereas Havelock Ellis tells us that Margaret, the Queen of Aragon, thought that six times a day was the correct number. Rubin reaches the conclusion that twice weekly was normal but that the American average was probably closer to once a week. Kinsey, on the other hand, dug up the information that it was three to four in youth and two to three in middle age — that is, weekly. But I am positive that Kinsey was way off base. About half his estimate would be closer to correct. So there it is. Who does know the answer?

Yet the authorities will go out on a limb and state that less than one-half of civilized men are blessed with normal sexual potency. I am forced to agree with this statement. In fact, I would go even a bit further and state that probably three men out of ten account for 70% of all sexual proclivity. What I am trying to say is that about three men out of ten indulge in sex three or four times weekly, whereas the other seven indulge in sex only two or three times monthly.

Here I would like to mention a rather important bit of information. I wonder just how many men know the difference between impotency and sterility. There is no similarity or connection between sterility and impotency. A man can be impotent and still be fertile or he can be sterile and not impotent. To take it further, a man may be fully capable of fertilizing a female and yet be impotent, whereas a man who has a high sexual output may be sterile. So the distinction is that potency refers only to the capacity to engage in sexual relations, whereas sterility is the inability, because of any one of many reasons, to discharge live sperm to impregnate the female.

There are also cases of partial impotency and complete impotency as well as permanent impotency and temporary impotency.

In dealing with the etiology of impotency, the following diseases can be contributing or causative factors: gonorrhea, syphilis, chronic obesity, mumps, stricture, meningitis, Bright's disease, diabetes, Addison's disease, myxoedema, orchitis, myelitis, cachexia and arteriosclerosis.

Most cases of impotency in men of forty and fifty are psychological. Speaking from actual experience as well as study, I give here some of the main factors that can influence psychological impotency: anxiety, fear of pregnancy, fear of discovery, a guilt complex, fear of venereal disease, fear of being unable to complete the act and revulsion caused by language or behaviour of the partner. While it may be suggested that some of these things are most trivial, yet I have found that they can, and do in many cases, cause temporary impotency. In the forefront I would place fear of being unable to perform the act or complete the act. The man who has learned to go to bed with his mate with a feeling of anticipation and with reckless, clearcut abandon will seldom fail to perform. But when he is keyed up or is seeking to make an impression or feels that there is an onus upon him, then the risk of failure looms realistically on the horizon.

You can depend upon it that once an inhibitory factor is found it may be impossible to rid oneself of it. I am sure that most males have already found that what I say here is absolutely true. As one writer put it, it is most highly probable that if a certain factor acted as an inhibitor on one occasion it can be counted upon to have a similar effect on every subsequent attempt at sexual intercourse with the same partner. When this happens to a single man it is of small consequence because he can readily change partners, but when this situation arises between a married man and his wife it can spell disaster for the marriage.

In facing the situation squarely, one realizes that the individual in most instances creates his own inhibitions. The higher the plane upon which the man places the sexual act or his partner, the greater the danger of finding or striking an inhibitory factor. If the male insists upon putting his female cohabitor on a pedestal or believes she is an angel or an idol or a gorgeous thing who is incapable of any deed or act or thought beyond the pale ... then

205

there is grave danger of finding that his idol has feet of clay. But if the male looks upon all females as females and thinks that they are all good, they are all nice, they are all beautiful, there is a good chance that he will have few inhibitions and seldom fail to perform promptly in the expected fashion.

I feel certain that you will understand that whereas a man might fail in his amorous attempts with his wife, the selfsame individual can readily perform in the arms of another female. Now this may not be according to Hoyle, it may be contrary to many people's concepts of right and decency, but here I am dealing with the topic of sex and I am speaking the truth even if it deviates somewhat from the accepted moral code.

There is an old standard joke about the woman who said to her husband, "Why, the lowly rooster can perform the sex act ten times a day!" And her husband replied, "Well, if I had a change of partners every time perhaps I could, too." There is more truth than poetry in that tale.

I suggest that if you are a pyjama-wearer that you discard them and let nature take its course. Perhaps you may be pleasantly surprised at the change that it will create in your sexual atmosphere. I contend that the wearing of pyjamas is not conducive to sexual potency.

## THE ART OF RETAINING SEXUAL VIRILITY INTO OLD AGE

If you are slipping, if you have lost your virility, if you are now impotent and are in the fifth or sixth or seventh decade of life, then the chance of making you virile and potent once again is, to say the least, rather remote ... but not entirely hopeless. I can hold out little promise for you.

However, all is not lost or forlorn — for there are natural, simple yet effective measures and means of regaining, maintaining or increasing the volume of sexual relations. I can find no reason why a man in good health cannot retain his sexual potency well into his 70's and

206

perhaps beyond. I can offer no magic, no potions, no aphrodisiacs, no drugs or preparations or concoctions.

However, returning to a natural form of living and eating can at least fully retain your present status and in most cases improve it and in my sincere opinion this is a distinct achievement well worth undertaking. If you will follow the rules of health as clearly indicated in this volume, your sexual relations should improve rather than decline. If you have managed to maintain sexual potency thus far, considering the conventional way you have been eating and living... then by changing your habits to conform to proper health standards, improvement will result without doubt.

Is it not clear and obvious that the lower the nutritional level of the body the lower the desire and the performance of sexual congress? I want to state here and now that there are no aphrodisiacal or passion foods. No, neither oysters nor honey nor raw eggs nor shell fish nor caviar nor mushrooms nor celery nor condiments nor pepper nor cinnamon nor milk and honey nor raw meat will perform the magic of making you sexually virile. However, and mark this well, good wholesome food as prescribed in this book will definitely function to maintain you in good health and as night follows day, better sexual relations will follow.

It has been known for centuries that the famed "Spanish-fly" or oil of cantharides is a powerful aphrodisiac. It is claimed that it definitely excites or irritates the sexual organs and glands, thus creating a demand for sexual relations. However, this is but a temporary measure and it can, in the long run, do more harm than good and its use is definitely not advised.

It is well to remember that when your eyesight or your hearing begin to fail, or when you begin to have stomach trouble or pancreatic malfunction or difficulty with any organ or function of the body, it is time to call a halt and take stock of yourself for the red light is flashing. This could clearly indicate faulty nutrition and if not corrected promptly it will result in or become a contributing factor towards sexual debility.

It would appear that primitive man had few or no sexual problems or difficulties and that the higher the culture or the civilization the lower the sexual potency. There is no room for doubt or conjecture . . . if we returned to nature and natural food and natural living, our sexual incidence would rise perceptibly. I have always suggested that man return to nature as closely as civilization will allow.

The rules of health advocated in this volume will create an atmosphere of well being, thus producing normal or high sexual frequency and a happy long life.

# CHAPTER 16

## Backache Banished

*Ignorance costs more than knowledge.*
.... W. A. ALCOTT, M.D.

### BACK TROUBLES

I have learned that there is one condition which seems to affect practically 100% of all the males in America. I don't know if this holds true in other parts of the world, but I suspect that it is also true in most of Europe. Here I am referring to males between the ages of 30 and 70 years.

It is said, and I have both heard and read it frequently, that human beings are heir to back trouble and that it cannot be avoided. They base their findings on the fact that all four legged animals except man walk on all fours and that because man walks upright which is contrary to the laws of gravity, he suffers backache. My answer to this contention is that it is nothing but a fairytale and no man need continue to suffer from this "back"affliction.

Now I am over sixty years of age and I distinctly recall suffering from back troubles intermittently ever since I was about 16 or 17 years old. This would mean that for over forty years I have had trouble with my back. And the trouble has ranged from minor discomfort to acute, insufferable agony.

I did recognize the fact that I would have my most severe attacks of back trouble in the spring and in the fall, but I attached little significance to this because of my occupation. I have been actively engaged in the nursery business for thirty-odd years and a nurseryman has his busiest periods in the spring and again in the fall. I attributed my back troubles mainly to the fact that as soon as the spring rush was over I got away from the fields and did my sedentary office work. Then when fall came along I would have to get active again and invariably about this time I'd have my "back attack" again. However, as soon as I got into the

209

swing of the heavy continuous physical labor, my back-aches ended. So I gathered it was either because I had long layoffs, allowing the muscles to become flabby, or because I lacked physical activity. Thus, when I started to work after a four month layoff, my unused back muscles became sore. That seemed to be a rational and reasonable explanation.

I did notice that the pains in my back and hip or as I referred to it, my "backaches" were becoming more severe with each succeeding year. To try to offset this, I began daily physical exercises and other activating chores of short duration throughout the entire year, with the hope that it would prevent the trouble when spring or fall came along. In other words, I was trying to keep my back muscles toned up all year. But this did not seem to prevent my backaches. I still had them as badly, yes, even worse than ever and this puzzled me no end because I figured that at last I had found a logical solution — that is, to maintain year-round muscle flexibility — and when I put it to the test, it failed me.

In March of 1960 I ran into a more than average attack of my back troubles and this time I swore that I would leave no stones unturned until I found the answer. This conviction was based on the assumption that somewhere I was doing something wrong or contrary to the laws of nature. I started by telling my wife that I would eat no more fish for a period. This went on for three or four days and I was not getting better. Actually I was getting worse! So I stopped eating meat to see if this would help, but to my horror, my condition became worse still. I gave up tea and coffee, I gave up using salt ... but still my condition was even more aggravated.

By now the pain and the suffering were more agonizing than I had ever known in my life. It was so bad now that I could not stand, I could not sit, I could not lie down and I could not sleep. I still continued my work at the office and if I sat down only for a few minutes, I could not get up again without help. When I got up in the morning I had to roll myself off the bed onto the floor and then gradually

210

raise myself up first on my elbows, then onto my knees and finally into a standing position.

I became bent over, leaning very heavily on my left side. My left leg began to bother me so much that no matter what position I was in I suffered untold agony. I can't even describe how horrible was the pain.

I clocked it on the calendar — I had not had more than an hour's sleep at a stretch in ten days.

I examined and scrutinized my diet. I could find absolutely nothing wrong with it. It seemed to be better than it had ever been. Still my condition worsened.

There was only one position that I could tolerate and that was walking. As long as I moved about I was in fairly comfortable circumstances. But when I stood still very long or sat down or got into bed, the pain was excrutiating.

I don't remember the exact day but somewhere around the 12th of March a man came in to see me. He introduced himself as Mr. Walker and said he'd like to talk to me for a moment. I invited him into my office and I eased myself into a chair as best I could and tried not to show my discomfort.

He informed me that he had read my book on Hunza and enjoyed it and just wanted to meet the man who wrote it . . . and being in this part of the country, he thought he'd drop in. So we chatted for about fifteen minutes and then he got up, held out his hand and said, "Mr. Tobe, I've taken enough of your time. I know you are a busy man and thank you for seeing me. Good-bye and good luck!"

We shook hands and he walked to the front door. I had followed after him and as he stood there with his hand on the knob, he looked up and saw a can of food that a young salesman of vegetarian foods had left me. It was marked Glutenburger.

He asked, "Do you have another moment to spare? I'd like to tell you something unusual."

I said, "Shoot . . . I'm listening!"

He went on, "That Glutenburger thing brought it to my mind."

"Maybe I didn't tell you," he said, "but I am in the

plaque business in Kitchener. My father started the business many years ago and I have continued it. Now in making plaques we use a paste made out of wheat."

"Why wheat specifically? I asked him.

"Well," he said, "we've tried most every known substance that can be used as paste or glue — the synthetics and the chemical ones and the plastics — but none of them are as good as plain ordinary wheat. They don't stand up as well as wheat and of course they are all much more expensive. All of these things are big factors in our production costs.

"However, using wheat has its disadvantages because every now and then things just go wrong. Through the years at various times the foreman or somebody from the factory would come in and say to my father or me, 'Everything has gone hay-wire again. I don't know what it is and I don't know what causes it, but the plaques are swelling up and breaking and nothing seems to be working right!'

"Now father had imparted to me that, strange to relate, this had been going on ever since he started using wheat paste to make these plaques stick together, but as this situation didn't happen every day and it only happened every now and then, he didn't pay too much attention to it. But when I became firmly interested in the business and accepted it as a career, I began to prepare charts. I don't know why I did it but I just did. Every time the foreman would report that the paste was acting up I'd make a note of the date. A few years went by and one day when things went really bad, I sat down and checked through my records. 'Twas then I realized that these troubles always arose in the spring or in the fall. I couldn't pin it down to March or April or October or November, but it was always in the spring and fall.

"This peculiar trouble did not take place during the entire spring or fall ... it just lasted a few days in each season. It could never be predicted nor did we know what the days would be, but it was during the seasonal periods of spring and fall. This struck me as being a phenomenon of nature. Even though the wheat was mutilated, had been

212

treated, was broken up and all that, there was something within it that began to act up in some mysterious way when spring or fall time came ... its normal time to grow."

He remained silent for a moment as though trying to solve something and then he went on, "That's my thought on the subject, but I'd like to get to the bottom of it. In fact, I have written to the agricultural college in Guelph to see if they know anything about it and if they have ever done any studies on the subject or if they can help me solve the mystery.

"As it stands now there is not much we can do about it. In fact, there is nothing we can do about it. But at least we know that come some time in the spring or some time in the fall we will have trouble with our paste. So we try to get most of our big batches and our most important work done during the troublefree months of the year."

When Mr. Walker had concluded that statement, he took his leave.

Suddenly a light or a flash went on in my brain. I looked up at the calendar — it was the 12th of March. I was leaning on a table and something made me remember a receipt that had come in the mail from a chiropractor to whom I had gone for treatment the previous fall. It was right under my hand, by some strange coincidence. I looked at it and there it was marked, "Three visits, November 4, 8 and 12."

"Why that's exactly when I have my back troubles," I said out loud. "That's when I've had my troubles all my life — in the spring and in the fall! Paste — wheat — my God, I have the answer!"

I regained my composure — though I really was excited — I went back into my office, shut the door, sat down, and carefully and deliberately began to think.

... This was the worst attack I'd ever known in my life. Then I recalled that through the years when I was but a child my father had suffered the same thing, only in his case it seemed to be much worse or more painful than mine because he used to scream. I vividly recall his actual screams because of the insufferable agony that he was going through. At those times I used to weep for my poor father.

213

The pain was so severe sometimes that he just couldn't stand it. My father was considered a very healthy man but at various times throughout the years he would suffer the agony of the damned because of his trouble with his back.

Then I said to myself, "A couple of weeks ago you gave up fish, and to make up for that you ate more bread. Then a few days later you gave up meat . . . and to make up for that deficiency, you ate more bread. Good gracious! Your diet the last ten days has consisted mostly of wheat products!

Well, from that moment on I ate no bread or any food containing wheat in any form. Within a few days after the elimination of all wheat products I was able to sleep. And then within a week my trouble was completely cleared up. This is true, so help me God!

On the 18th day of March I went to New York to the flower show. I was not completely free of pain but I was in good enough condition to travel and drive my car. I hadn't missed the flower show in many years and I didn't want to miss this one . . . although a few days prior I had given up the prospect of going, due to my agonizing condition.

Five years have elapsed since that episode and I have never had a recurrence of my trouble. At times I do get a warning and when I get a twinge in my back or in my left leg, I immediately cut down or completely eliminate bread and all other wheat products from my diet for a few days or a week.

I have passed this information on to various friends of mine. Some have believed me and tried it and have told me that it has worked for them just as well as it did for me. Others wouldn't try it . . . and they still have their back troubles. In every case where it has been given a fair trial it has brought the predicted results.

To be most effective all wheat products must be strictly eliminated for at least four or five days or better still, for a week or longer. Exercise or physical labor in keeping with your strength and capabilities should be undertaken. The more energy you burn up the sooner you will get over your back troubles.

To me this information and knowledge came at my most desperate period . . . yes, I consider that it came at the most crucial moment of my life.

If you suffer from back troubles, I beg of you, in fact, I plead with you to try abstaining from anything that contains wheat for four or five days.

This does not mean that you have to abstain from ever eating wheat again. You just lay off when you run into trouble or when you get a warning of impending complications. You will learn to detect it just as I have learned to detect it. You will get a sharp twinge of pain in the muscles of your back or one or both legs will begin to hurt or stiffen. If that happens, lay off anything that contains wheat.

There appears to be little doubt that in the Western world we eat too much wheat in various forms. One writer in Britain estimated that in that country wheat products comprise up to 60% of the total food intake. I do not believe it is that high in America but I would assume that it would run at least 25% to 40% of the bulk intake . . . and that is definitely too much wheat or any other one food.

Now this is all not as nonsensical as you may believe or think. Since that time, from my studies, my observations, my searchings, I have found the rhyme and the reason . . . and here it is. I found it in a book called *Basic Nutrition and Cell Nutrition* by R. F. Milton, B.Sc., Ph.D., F.R.I.C. and I will quote from this book:

"The second main enzyme in pancreatic juice is amylase. It is similar to the ptyalin of the saliva in that its function is to break down starches to simple sugars. The ptyalin has partially broken down the starches to dextrins, and the amylases in the small intestine continue with the digestion to produce sugars of simple molecular size. With certain starches, e.g., wheat, the dextrin first breaks down to maltose; it is then acted upon by an amylase enzyme known as maltase which results in the production of glucose units. These are small enough to pass across the intestine membrane into the blood stream. They then pass into the liver where they are converted into human starch (glycogen) by a similar enzyme and so stored until required."

215

It appears that the body uses wheat and wheat products for making glycogen. Now there are many other foods from which the body can and does make glycogen but wheat seems to be the most important one or the easiest one. In any event, whatever the means or the method, wheat triggers it or is in itself the culprit. But the clear fact is that the body does use wheat to make glycogen . . . and most of us eat more wheat than we do any other individual food.

The body stores glycogen in the liver. When the liver is filled up, the body begins to store the glycogen in your muscles and that is where your trouble begins. As soon as you stop eating wheat and become active, the body utilizes the glycogen from your muscles and your troubles are soon over. Exercise or physical labor evidently utilizes or burns up the glycogen and relief follows. People who do heavy physical work can stand lots of bread and other wheat products; but for those who are not active, bread and other wheat products can cause trouble.

You can check this knowledge about glycogen with your doctor, with any scientist, with a biochemist or with whomever you want to check it, or in any good biochemical textbook, and you'll find the information given above to be true.

Now lest you think that just be eliminating bread your troubles are over, I want to warn you that they will not be over because wheat is present in many foods where it is not recognized. Many processors use wheat as a filler because wheat is among the best of foods for this purpose. Wheat is a wholesome food and, best and happiest of all, wheat is one of the cheapest foods on earth. It only costs the processors about 2¢ or 3¢ a pound at the most. That is why they use wheat in so many processed foods.

Now maybe you don't know it and would never suspect it but chocolate bars contain a good proportion of wheat. You see, wheat tastes good and it picks up the flavor of the chocolate well and is also a good bulking agent . . . and of course, as I mentioned before, it is about the cheapest of all foods.

Now I'm going to give you a list of some of the common

216

foods that contain wheat so that when you make an attempt to avoid eating wheat to prevent that backache, you will know what to guard against. Bread (any kind of bread, because almost invariably rye, oatmeal, soya and other breads contain 20% to 60% wheat anyway), cakes, pies, cookies, doughnuts, biscuits, shortbreads and all baked goods, stews, postum and other burnt cereal beverages, chocolates, macaroni, spaghetti, noodles, chow mein, breaded meats and fish, cereals and other foods that contain wheat and with which I am not familiar.

Here I'd also like to state that not every backache is caused by the condition I mentioned — that is, the glycogen factor derived from wheat — but I'll wager that nine out of ten cases will clear up easily and quickly by the mere abstinence from wheat or any food or product that contains wheat.

## WHAT YOU SHOULD KNOW ABOUT WHEAT

In the Americas wheat is king. In Europe rye and barley are of greater economic importance. In Asia, rice is the most important of all of the foods. Rice, of course, is also the most important single food in the world because there are more Asians than there are other people, and they prefer rice.

Wheat contains a splendidly balanced combination of all the vital elements in the form of proteins, carbohydrates and fats. It is my belief that the balance of proteins, carbohydrates and fats in wheat is as close to perfect as it is possible to obtain.

Its economic importance cannot be exaggerated, for its low price and abundance make it the most vital of all foods for people living in the temperate zones. I believe it is the lowest priced food obtainable in America, if not in the world.

Many years ago it had been estimated that one day's normal labor on a wheat farm with modern tillage and harvesting equipment can provide the food requirements of one person for an entire year.

217

Now I'd like to mention that while I consider wheat one of the finest of foods, yet the condition and the form in which it reaches you, the consumer, it is not only a devitalized, poor food but can even be decidedly harmful. As you undoubtedly know, wheat as such is seldom included in the diet of any people throughout the world. After being milled it is still seldom utilized in its whole form with its components intact. Invariably, when we eat wheat we get it in the form of bread, pies, cakes, cookies, biscuits, spaghetti, cream of wheat, cereals and other forms and it has been treated, heated, fractioned, fragmented, until it would be next to impossible to recognize it for what it was originally.

From the time it is processed in the mill till the time that it reaches the consumer the changes that it undergoes, including the many chemical additives that are mixed with it, make it no longer a food but turn it into a vile, vicious, detrimental chemical concoction. Whether or not you know it, it is a fact that there are approximately twenty-five different chemicals that can be and are added to wheat and bread. Here I list these chemicals as quoted from the official Food and Drug Act and Regulations . . .

1. Oxides of nitrogen
2. Chlorine
3. Chlorine dioxide
4. Nitrosyl chloride
5. Benzoyl peroxide
6. Calcium carbonate
7. Calcium sulphate
8. Dicalcium phosphate
9. Magnesium carbonate
10. Potassium aluminum sulphate
11. Sodium aluminum sulphate
12. Tricalcium phosphate
13. Potassium bromate
14. Ammonium persulphate
15. Ammonium chloride
16. Calcium lactate
17. Diammonium phosphate

218

18. Monoammonium phosphate
19. Potassium iodide
20. Monocalcium phosphate
21. Potassium iodate
22. Calcium peroxide
23. Potassium persulphate
24. Propionic acid
25. Sodium diacetate
26. Sorbic acid
   Plus a wide variety of chemical food colors, including *arsenic.*

I would further like to make it clear at this point that the harm that results from the eating of wheat products is not necessarily the fault of the wheat but the fault first of fragmentation and secondly, the chemical additives that it contains.

Take this one statement from an important book on nutrition: "Finely milled flour is greatly superior in keeping qualities to the whole grain." Of course it is superior in keeping qualities for it is "dead" because all of the germ and practically all of the bran are discarded. There you have the crux of the situation ... the keeping qualities or shelf-life are far more important in our economy than the health and the well-being of the people.

Wheat is an annual or biennial grass, properly known as Triticum sativum. It is believed by some authorities to be the first of the grains domesticated by man and its cultivation, they suggest, began in the Neolithic period. Because wheat thrives best in the cool weather it is grown chiefly in the temperate regions of the world.

The great wheat-producing countries of the world are the United States, China, Russia, Canada, Argentina and Australia. It is indeed a pity that wheat which is one of nature's great contributions to the welfare of mankind has been so horribly defiled and corrupted to the state where it now causes mankind more pains and diseases than any other food.

# CHAPTER 17

## Menus and Recipes

*"Many people just simply are not aware of the fact that what they eat, or do not eat, has a profound influence on their health."*

: : : . DR. W. H. SEBRELL, JR.

### MENUS FOR A MONTH

In the preparation of this book I had not intended to assume the guise of a dietician or cook. However, I received repeated proddings from friends, acquaintances, critics, and readers who said in essence, "By your teaching and admonitions you are depriving us of all the foods that we like, that are readily available and acceptable and to which we are accustomed, so at least suggest something in their place!"

This argument was so reasonable and pointed that I felt I had no recourse — I just had to prepare a menu and selection of recipes.

So here are the suggested menus for thirty-one days.

1. Breakfast — Big slice melon
   Lunch — Sandwich, cole slaw, herb tea
   Dinner — Big vegetable salad, baked potato, cheese
2. Breakfast — 10 oz. citrus juice
   Lunch — Raw vegetable salad & Flahonse
   Dinner — Casserole, fruit and nuts
3. Breakfast — Bowl of Muesli
   Lunch — Fruits in season & nuts (3 oz.)
   Dinner — Big vegetable salad, rice risotto
4. Breakfast — 10 oz. mixed vegetable juice
   Lunch — Raw vegetable salad & Flahonse
   Dinner — Soup, baked potato, fruit
5. Breakfast — Bowl of prunes
   Lunch — Fruits in season & nuts (3 oz.)
   Dinner — Big vegetable salad, Spanish rice, cheese
6. Breakfast — 10 oz. carrot juice
   Lunch — Raw vegetable salad & Flahonse
   Dinner — Casserole, fruit and nuts

7. Breakfast — Apricots and raisins
   Lunch — Sandwich and small salad
   Dinner — Soup, big vegetable salad, cheese
8. Breakfast — Big slice melon
   Lunch — Sandwich, cole slaw, herb tea
   Dinner — Big vegetable salad, baked potato, cheese
9. Breakfast — 10 oz. citrus juice
   Lunch — Raw vegetable salad & Flahonse
   Dinner — Casserole, fruit, nuts
10. Breakfast — Bowl of Muesli
    Lunch — Fruits in season & nuts (3 oz.)
    Dinner — Vegetable salad, soy bean dish, herb tea
11. Breakfast — 10 oz. mixed vegetable juice
    Lunch — Raw vegetable salad & Flahonse
    Dinner — Soup, baked potato, fruit
12. Breakfast — Bowl of prunes
    Lunch — Fruits in season & nuts (3 oz.)
    Dinner — Big vegetable salad, vegetable chop suey
13. Breakfast — 10 oz. carrot juice
    Lunch — Raw vegetable salad & Flahonse
    Dinner — Casserole, fruit, nuts
14. Breakfast — Figs
    Lunch — Sandwich, small salad
    Dinner — Big vegetable salad, soup, cheese
15. Breakfast — Big slice melon
    Lunch — Sandwich, cole slaw, herb tea
    Dinner — Big vegetable salad, baked potato, cheese
16. Breakfast — 10 oz. citrus juice
    Lunch — Raw vegetable salad & Flahonse
    Dinner — Casserole, fruit and nuts
17. Breakfast — Bowl of Muesli
    Lunch — Fruits in season & nuts (3 oz.)
    Dinner — Big vegetable salad, brown rice loaf
18. Breakfast — 10 oz. mixed vegetable juice
    Lunch — Raw vegetable salad & Flahonse
    Dinner — Soup, baked potato, fruit
19. Breakfast — Bowl of prunes
    Lunch — Fruits in season & nuts (3 oz.)
    Dinner — Big vegetable salad, Spanish pancakes

20. Breakfast — 10 oz. carrot juice
    Lunch — Raw vegetable salad & Flahonse
    Dinner — Casserole and fruit and nuts

21. Breakfast — Peaches and raisins
    Lunch — Sandwich and small salad
    Dinner — Big vegetable salad, soup, cheese

22. Breakfast — Big slice melon
    Lunch — Sandwich, cole slaw, herb tea
    Dinner — Big vegetable salad, baked potato, cheese

23. Breakfast — 10 oz. citrus juice
    Lunch — Raw vegetable salad & Flahonse
    Dinner — Casserole, fruit, nuts

24. Breakfast — Bowl of Muesli
    Lunch — Fruits in season & nuts (3 oz.)
    Dinner — Big vegetable salad, buckwheat Spanish
        style

25. Breakfast — 10 oz. mixed vegetable juice
    Lunch — Raw vegetable salad & Flahonse
    Dinner — Soup, baked potato, fruit

26. Breakfast — Bowl of prunes
    Lunch — Fruits in season & nuts (3 oz.)
    Dinner — Big vegetable salad, steamed brown rice

27. Breakfast — 10 oz. carrot juice
    Lunch — Raw vegetable salad & Flahonse
    Dinner — Casserole, fruit and nuts

28. Breakfast — Apricots and raisins
    Lunch — Sandwich, small salad
    Dinner — Soup, big vegetable salad, cheese

29. Breakfast — Big slice melon
    Lunch — Raw vegetable salad & Flahonse
    Dinner — Big vegetable salad, baked potato, cheese

30. Breakfast — 10 oz. citrus juice
    Lunch — Raw vegetable salad & Flahonse
    Dinner — Casserole, fruit and nuts

31. Breakfast — Bowl of Muesli
    Lunch — Bananas or berries and nuts, herb tea
    Dinner — Big vegetable salad, millet Spanish style

I firmly and emphatically contend that the best, the foremost diet for man is the mono-diet... that is, one food for each meal. Realizing that a mono-diet would be most monotonous — especially for those of us who have been trained to eat three or four or many more foods at one meal — in my suggested menu I include more than one food at each meal, except breakfast. But common sense and study will reveal that the best diet is the mono-diet and this could be a goal for the future.

Make sure you do not eat the same vegetable every day. Strive for variety, not necessarily at every meal but every day.

At this time I would like to make it clear and positive that I do not recommend or permit the use of cooked foods in the optimum diet... but recognizing the frailties of human nature, I would suggest that if you must partake of cooked foods that you do it only at one meal a day, preferably the evening meal. Even then, only part of your meal is to consist of cooked foods. Optimum health cannot be obtained from cooked foods, even if lightly cooked. Heating above 120 degrees kills enzymes.

If you must eat cooked foods, I consider soups among the best for the minerals are not leached out and lost. However, whether or not your body can assimilate them is another question.

*Cooked Foods Permitted* — Baked potatoes, sweet potatoes, beets, squash, apples, rice, millet, buckwheat, steamed whole onions, carrots, eggplant, oatmeal, a casserole consisting of various vegetables.

All juices must be fresh — never canned, bottled or frozen.

Where citrus juices are given you may instead have 3 or 4 oranges or whole grapefruit.

The 10 oz. of fruit or vegetable juice should be ample and you should try to make it do, but if you are hungry add 2 oz. Muesli.

Melons mentioned may be watermelon, muskmelon, honeydew, Spanish or others.

If desired, have clabber or yoghurt with your vegetable salad, but not more than 3 times weekly. Be sure it is made from fresh, whole, unpasteurized milk.

Vegetable juices are advised over fruit juices.

Other fruit juices are advised over citrus juices.

No foods containing chemical additives are to be used anywhere along with this menu.

Monosodium glutamate is totally and unequivocally forbidden.

Salt in any form, including iodized, should be avoided but if it must be used, use sea salt or natural salt in limited quantities.

Baking soda and baking powder are positively forbidden.

Glucose, white sugar and other synthetic or fragmented sweeteners are forbidden.

I do not recommend the use of any processed product for flavoring, strengthening or seasoning anything. The vegetables themselves, along with the best oil that you can procure and culinary herbs, should give you the finest seasoned soup available.

Use leaf or Romaine lettuce wherever possible. The tight head lettuce is the poorest.

I recommend the use of onions and garlic in spite of the fact that many nutritionists suggest you avoid their use. My studies reveal that they are not harmful but actually beneficial.

Sprouts are good food and should be included in the daily diet, especially for those living in the northern latitudes and during the winter when fresh vegetables are not readily available.

When making salads, use the vegetables or fruits as whole as possible. This is generally referred to as a finger salad. The more you chop or grind the fruit or vegetable, the greater the nutritional loss. I have found that when you get used to eating them whole you will not want them cut, chopped or grated.

If you must have a beverage use a herb tea or fresh,

home-made juices — never tea, coffee or alcoholic beverages. Another palatable beverage is a hot or cold, preferably cold, mixture of unpasteurized cider vinegar, honey and water. Mix a teaspoonful of honey, 2 teaspoonsful of vinegar and add water to taste. This makes a very pleasant refreshing drink.

Breads of any kind — even the best home-made ones — are not, according to my knowledge, good food. Admittedly, they are very filling and satisfying and I condone their use, especially when someone is struggling to change his diet. But eventually they will be found to be totally unnecessary. Always make sure that your breads are made from untreated whole grains, be they wheat, rye, soya or others.

I do not advocate the use of flesh food or fish or even eggs or milk in any form. This is a difficult admission for me to make because I was accustomed, all my life until past fifty, to a largely flesh food or carnivorous diet. However, my studies have made the conventional diet untenable. I could not ignore the overwhelming proof that presented itself. So I suggest to you that you avoid the use of meats, fish and all animal products.

I also urge you to use no processed foods. There never was and never will be a processed food that is fit food for a human being.

Learn to use a wider variety of raw vegetables . . . yes, raw asparagus, beets, beet tops, broccoli, endive, peas, mushrooms, potatoes, parsley, parsnips, spinach, turnips, Chinese radish and many others. In fact, the whole vegetable kingdom can be used raw — even most grasses. I know the delight I found when I first ate beets raw. I could hardly believe my sense of taste because they are so pleasant and sweet. The same applies to many other vegetables.

I would avoid the use of cashews. While they are a very pleasant and tasty nut, they invariably come in cans and have been treated with some kind of gas as well as having been processed and therefore I cannot consider them a live, satisfactory food.

Always use fruits, grains of vegetables as nearly ripe as possible. In my opinion unripe foods such as bananas, avocados, tomatoes, melons, papayas, cucumbers, squash and many others are not nearly as good or as nutritious as the same food when ripened. I think we all understand that in the ripening process chemical changes take place in the food and as we want the full benefits from our food, I think they should be allowed to ripen as much as possible . . . that is, let them ripen well but eat them before they get rotten.

Let us stress here that if you followed the best diet in the world and persisted in drinking alcoholic beverages and smoking cigarettes and guzzling soft drinks, you would definitely not be able to maintain good health. I repeat . . . if you indulge in these degenerative practices, then good health is impossible.

At this point I would also like to make it clear that I do not believe there are any such things as miracle foods, health foods or curative foods. All of nature's blessed bounties are beneficial in balance and as nature made them.

## SALADS

### Vegetable Salad (All Raw)

Cut string beans, young okra, mustard greens, chicory, watercress, red onion, carrots, Romaine lettuce, escarole, Bibb lettuce, celery, green peppers, tomatoes, watercress, etc. Toss with soya oil, herbs and lemon juice.

### Slaw Salad

Slired cabbage finely, add shredded carrots for flavor and streaking. A dash of lemon juice or apple cider vinegar will add piquancy.

## Cabbage Combination Salad

1 cup chopped or shredded cabbage
½ cup grated carrot
½ cup grated beet
½ cup minced celery
2 tablespoons minced parsley

2 tablespoons chopped green onion

Mix all ingredients well and blend with homemade French dressing.

## Mabel's Salad

2 cups chopped cabbage
½ cup sliced radish
½ cup chopped bell pepper
½ cup chopped tomato
½ cup chopped green onion
3 tablespoons minced parsley

Blend all ingredients well together and mix with homemade French dressing or mayonnaise.

## Bean Sprout Salad

2 cups bean sprouts
½ cup chopped celery
½ cup chopped tomato
½ cup minced green onion

Mix well with homemade French dressing.

## Lettuce-Celery Salad

1 cup chopped lettuce
1 cup chopped celery
½ cup chopped bell pepper

Mix together and add homemade French dressing.

## Lettuce-Watercress Salad

2 cups chopped lettuce
1 cup chopped watercress
Mix with French dressing.

## Combination Salad I

3 parts chopped lettuce to 1 part each sliced radishes, chopped tomato and minced parsley. Moisten with French dressing.

## Combination Salad II

3 parts chopped lettuce to 1 part each of chopped celery, chopped sweet green pepper, chopped tomato, and minced green onion to flavor, if desired. Mix with French dressing.

## Asparagus Salad

Equal parts asparagus and watercress tips. Place layer of each in salad bowl, then a layer of sliced tomato. Drip French dressing over it.

## Brilliant Salad

6 beet leaves
¼ lb. cabbage
¼ avocado (in season)
1 carrot
1 sliced tomato
1 stalk celery with tops
Parsley to flavor

Mix finely cut beet leaves and shredded cabbage together. Mince celery and parsley, grate carrot, and add avocado and sliced tomato. Serve with or without dressing. Serves one.

## Variety Salad

1 small head fresh green lettuce
4 ripe tomatoes
1 green pepper
1 large onion
1 medium cucumber
1 cup fresh crisp spinach
Few sprigs of fresh watercress or parsley

Cut lettuce into quarters. Cut rest of ingredients and mix. Serve on beet leaves with sprig of watercress or parsley. Season with fresh lime or lemon juice or your favorite dressing. Serves four.

## Relish Salad

2 cups finely chopped cabbage
1 grated onion
½ cup chopped beets
1 cup minced celery

3 tbs. minced pimento
½ minced green pepper

Mix with your favorite dressing. Serves three.

### Simple Salad

½ head fresh cabbage
2 carrots
1 green pepper
1 stalk celery
1 onion

Grate cabbage and carrots. Dice pepper, celery, onion and mix all vegetables together. May be served with lemon juice or a sprinkling of grated nuts.

### Quick Salad

1 cup chopped dandelion leaves
1 cup chopped chicory or Chinese cabbage
½ bunch chopped beet tops
½ head chopped green lettuce
½ cup chopped spinach
½ cup chopped watercress

Mix all vegetables together and serve with lemon juice and honey. Add a sprinkling of grated or chopped nuts.

### Satisfaction Salad

¼ medium head green crisp cabbage
1 medium or 2 small beets

2 small carrots
2 ripe tomatoes
1 medium cucumber or 2 small ones
1 medium green pepper

Grate cabbage, carrots and beets. Slice cucumber. Cut pepper into rings. Slice or quarter tomatoes. Arrange cabbage, carrots and beets in individual mounds on leaves. Surround by slices of cucumber. Place rings of pepper and tomatoes on top. Place stalk of celery on the side and serve.

### Tasty Salad

1 cup shredded cabbage
1 grated carrot
6 ripe olives
1 clove of garlic
½ cup diced green pepper
½ cup diced celery

Rub a clove of garlic on salad bowl and toss in all the vegetables. Cut in olives and mix well. Add your favorite dressing.

### Cole Slaw

1 small head green cabbage
3 stalks celery
2 large carrots
1 large green pepper
¾ cup finely cut parsley

Wash and grate vegetables. Make dressing of 2 tbsp. oil and juice of one lemon. Pour over vegetables and mix thoroughly.

### Crunchy Salad

½ small green cabbage
1 stalk celery
2 sweet apples
¼ lb. shelled nuts

Chop together and serve with a border of watercress, escarole or chicory. Flavor with lemon juice, if desired, before serving, or any other favorite dressing.

### Eggplant Salad

1 good-sized eggplant
2 stalks green celery
2 large or 3 small green peppers
2 medium onions

Bake eggplant in skin. Peel and mash in wooden bowl with wooden spoon. Chop celery, peppers and onions, add to eggplant and mix thoroughly. Serve on lettuce leaves. For dressing add lemon or lime juice.

### Avocado Tomato Salad

½ avocado
4 tomatoes

1 pepper
2 stalks celery
1 onion

Dice celery, pepper and onion. Add mashed avocado and mix. Scoop out tomato pulp, cut fine and add to mixture. Add lemon juice. Fill tomatoes and serve.

### Yogurt Dream Salad

3 radishes
½ cucumber
½ green pepper
2 scallions
3 oz. pot cheese
½ glass yogurt or clabbered milk

Dice all vegetables, add pot cheese and yogurt. A few leaves of watercress, cut up, goes well with this.

If cucumber is scarce substitute shredded green squash (zucchini).

### Berry-Fruit Salad

2 tbs. raspberries
2 tbs. blueberries
3 tbs. watermelon balls
3 tbs. muskmelon balls
1 ripe banana

Place fruit on crisp lettuce leaves. Place slices of banana around it. Serve with pineapple juice and honey.

## Tasty Fruit Salad

1 pear
1 peach
1 apple
½ cup grapes

Slice the fruits, halve the grapes, and mix. Serve on lettuce leaves with nuts and honey.

## Waldorf Salad

½ cup shredded green cabbage
½ cup shredded green celery
1 cup finely shredded apple
½ cup seedless raisins
¼ cup shredded nuts

Mix and serve on green lettuce leaves. If dressing is desired, use one-half ripe mashed avocado. Add lemon juice if desired.

# SALAD DRESSINGS

## French Dressing

¾ cup tomato juice
1 or 2 tbs. soy oil

Juice of ⅓ lemon
Half clove of garlic or a little grated onion.

Shake well before serving.

### Simplicity Dressing

Into a cold bowl put 3 tablespoons vegetable oil. Add 2 tablespoons of lemon juice, 1 tablespoon each of onion juice and finely minced parsley and a dash of paprika. Beat well.

### Oil and Lemon Dressing

Soy oil and lemon juice, well blended, or whipped with a fork.

### Special French Dressing

Olive oil, lemon juice and honey — equal parts.

### Special Dressing

Mix 2 tbs. milk or cream, 2 tbs. honey, 3 tbs. salad oil, juice of ½ lemon, 2 cloves of garlic, mashed well.

## Herbal Salad Dressing for Vegetables

Combine 2 tablespoons olive oil, 2 teaspoons fresh lemon juice, 1 teaspoon cream, and a dash of honey — about as much as the tip of a teaspoon will hold. Add 1 teaspoon finely grated onion, a smidgin of mashed garlic and some finely cut chives and parsley. When available, add other finely cut, fresh aromatic herbs such as thyme, marjoram, tarragon, borage, mint, etc. In winter, frozen or dried herbs are good additions.

## SOUPS

### Vegetable Soup

Put 1 tomato, 1 carrot, 1 small pepper, 1 stalk celery, 1 small apple, 1 ounce almonds, and ½ cup wheat flakes through fine vegetable grinder.

Add milk to taste, allowing to stand an hour or two. Heat gently, stirring in ½ cup of thick cream (do not boil); serve.

### Bean and Barley Soup

¼ cup small white beans
¼ cup garbanzo beans
¼ cup soy beans
¼ cup small lima beans
¼ cup barley
2 large onions
3 - 4 cloves garlic, mashed

4 quarts water
3 large stalks celery with leaves, diced
2 large carrots, diced
1 large parsnip, diced
3 - 4 tablespoons sunflower oil
5 fresh mushrooms, sliced
1 tablespoon powdered kelp
Pinch of oregano, sweet basil and rosemary

Soak beans and barley overnight in water to cover, saving water they were soaked in. Sauté onions in oil. Add beans and barley and a total of 4 quarts water. Cook for one hour. Add vegetables, herbs, and kelp. Cook for one more hour.

### Vegetable Soup (unfired)

1 cup chopped carrots
1 cup chopped celery
1 cup fresh peas
½ cup asparagus pieces
2 tomatoes, cut in small pieces
1 chopped onion
2 sprigs parsley, chopped

Place 1 quart water on fire to boil. Meanwhile, combine all vegetable ingredients in large bowl. Pour boiling water over mixture, but do not cook. Allow to set until soup is cool enough to consume.

For variations, 2 cups tomato juice may be used to replace 2 cups water, adding the juice after it has been warmed but not boiled. Turnips, potatoes, spinach, okra, string beans, or other vegetables, may be used to replace one-half of vegetables in basic recipe.

## Cream of Celery Soup

Steam celery and celery tops with an onion. Pour celery and its juice into blender and blend. Add vegetable oil and herbs while still blending. Strain, add sweet basil, chopped parsley. The same style of soup can be made as above with varying ingredients such as carrots, peas, green pepper, tomatoes and herbs.

## Cereal Soup

Soak 10 oz. oatmeal in warm water overnight. Add 1 cup each tomato juice and pulp and chopped celery. Flavor with 3 tablespoons finely minced parsley and grated or whole onion, or a clove of very finely minced and crushed garlic instead of the onion to suit your taste. This may be varied by substituting kernels of tender corn, scraped from the cob, for the celery.

## Beet Soup

Liquefy cooked whole beets. Add lemon juice to taste and a little raw sugar or honey if desired.

Serve hot or cold. Yogurt or clabbered milk may be added.

## Lentil Soup

    2 cups lentils (soaked)
    3 carrots
    1 green pepper
    ½ head celery

Dice carrots, celery and pepper. Mix vegetables and lentils. Add 6 cups water. Bring to a boil and simmer for 30 minutes.

### Onion Soup

2 large onions
1 large carrot
1 green pepper
½ cup parsley
½ cup brown rice (steamed)

Bring 6 cups of water to a boil. Dice carrot, pepper and onions. Mix with brown rice and put mixture into boiling water. Simmer for 30 minutes.

### Potato Soup

6 small potatoes
1 onion
2 stalks celery
1 carrot

Dice all vegetables. Add 3 cups water. Bring to boil and simmer for 30 minutes. Serve with a sprinkling of parsley greens.

### Tomato Soup

8 tomatoes
1 bunch parsley
1 onion

Pour 6 cups of water over tomatoes and onions. Bring to boil and simmer for 10 minutes. Strain through coarse strainer, discarding the skins. Cut or chop parsley and sprinkle over soup. Add lemon juice, if desired.

### Consommé Végétal

2 carrots of medium size
1 turnip
1 stalk of leek
2 onions
2 tablespoonfuls of rice
1 tablespoonful of barley
4 tablespoonfuls of oil
2 quarts of water

Combine and bring to boil, then let simmer covered for 45 minutes. Season with kelp. It will then be ready for use. Break an egg into a bowl and pour the hot broth of your soup over the egg. As soon as you see the white of the egg cooked, stir up the yolk, and let it mix with the broth. If you desire you may sprinkle a little green parsley over the broth.

### Unfired Asparagus and Celery Soup

½ cup water
8 stalks asparagus
Top of celery — 1 stalk
½ small onion
Rosemary
Sunflower seeds
Kelp to season

Chop fine or mix in blender. Add further seasoning if desired.

## Unfired Cabbage and Beet Soup

½ cup water
2 cabbage leaves
1 beet and top
½ small onion
15 raisins
1 slice lemon with rind
Oregano
Pepper

Chop fine or mix in blender. Add further seasoning if desired.

# MAIN COURSE DISHES

## Eggplant Casserole

Cut eggplant into cubes (with skin), put into pan, add peeled sliced onion, chopped celery tops, green pepper, diced and fresh quartered ripe tomatoes. Add enough water to keep bottom from burning. Start on high heat until it begins to cook, then turn down low and let simmer for 15 minutes.

Put about half of these vegetables through blender with

vegetable oil to taste. Pour back blended vegetables into steamed ones and mix together. If you wish, you may also add chunks of peeled fresh tomatoes and sprinkle with oregano.

Any fresh vegetables may be treated in the same way. Yellow squash is good, but omit tomatoes.

### Casserole of Baby Lima Beans

Put 1 cup baby lima beans into pan with sliced tomato, sliced celery, sliced carrots, chopped onions, a pinch of sweet basil and other herbs and a dash of vegetable oil. Add a little water, cook for 15 minutes.

### Broccoli Casserole

Steam broccoli for 15 minutes. While this is steaming, brown 1 clove chopped garlic and herbs, add juice of half a lemon, then put broccoli into a baking pan. Sprinkle grated natural Swiss or cheddar cheese on top and brown slightly under broiler.

### Millet

Overnight soak 1 cup millet seeds in 2 cups water. Cook same as rice and during last 10 minutes add marjoram or oregano and garlic. Add vegetable oil before serving.

## Spanish Buckwheat

2 cups boiling water
1 tsp. kelp
1 cup whole buckwheat

Add buckwheat and kelp to boiling water and boil for 20 minutes on medium flame. Add sauce to cereal and bake in covered casserole in 350° oven for 1 hour.

## Spanish Sauce

3 medium onions
¼ lb. mushrooms
1 green pepper
¼ cup sunflower oil
1 large tomato
1 tsp. paprika
½ tsp. ground pepper
1½ tsps. kelp

Dice onions, add oil and sauté for 5 minutes, add cut mushrooms, continue to sauté for another 5 minutes. Add diced green pepper and sliced tomato and seasoning. Sauté all for 15 minutes more on low flame.

## Spanish Rice

2 cups boiling water
1 tsp. kelp
1 cup brown rice

Add brown rice and kelp to boiling water and boil for 20 min. on medium flame. Add sauce to cereal and bake in covered casserole in 350° oven for 1 hour.

## Vegetable Stew

1 medium sized eggplant
2 zucchini squash
2 onions
½ green or red pepper
3 fresh tomatoes
2 carrots
1 stalk celery
1 cup shelled peas

Dice all ingredients except the peas.

Sauté onion and peppers in 2 tbs. soya oil until soft (not brown), add tomatoes and steam for 15 minutes. Add ½ cup water, 1 tsp. herbs and the balance of the vegetables. Steam for 25 minutes.

## Rice Risotto

Boil 2 cups water, add 1 cup brown rice and 2 large pinches of dried mushrooms, and let simmer for 40 minutes. While waiting, steam carrots, peas, celery and green peppers. Put a little vegetable oil in a deep serving dish, add rice and the above vegetables and mix.

## Soya Bean Dish

Soak overnight 1 cup soya beans in 2 cups water. Next day add enough water to cover and simmer for about 30 minutes. Add shredded onion, 2 sliced carrots and cook for 15 minutes. Add tomatoes, celery, herbs and a dash of powdered kelp or dulse and cook for 5 minutes more.

## Mitzie's Casserole

    1 clove garlic
    1 green pepper
    2 onions, cut fine
    ¼ lb. mushrooms (if desired)

Put in skillet with a tablespoon of oil for one minute
only. Then remove from heat.

Into casserole put
    ¼ eggplant, skin and all
        Broccoli, cut in large pieces
    1 large yam or squash
    2 stalks Chinese greens
    2 sliced zucchini, skin and all
    Asparagus, cut in large pieces
    2 kohlrabi
    4 water chestnuts (optional)

Put half of ingredients into casserole, then put in 1 tablespoon ground herb mixture, 1 tablespoon ground dulse.
Cover with onion and green pepper mixture and then remaining half of vegetables. Slice tomatoes in ¼ to ½ inch
thickness over top. Put into pre-heated oven of 400 degrees
for 20 minutes only. Do not over-bake.

## Simple Muesli

    2 tablespoons coarse rolled oats
    1 tablespoon lemon juice
    1 cup chopped apple
    1 tablespoon honey
    ½ cup milk
    1 tablespoon nut meats

Soak rolled oats in milk for 30 minutes. Add other ingredients and mix well. Chill in refrigerator and serve cold.

For variation, use grated apple or mashed berries instead of chopped apple, or use cream instead of milk. Finely grated nut meats may be sprinkled on Muesli if desired.

## Steamed Brown Rice

Sauté cut-up onions and garlic in olive, sunflower, corn or soya oil until slightly browned. Add cut-up celery stalks and some of the leaves. Add hot water to cover. Steam for 10 minutes. Add washed brown rice and mix well after adding enough hot water to thoroughly cover. Steam another ½ hour or until done. No salt or pepper is used.

When serving, add a large pat of butter to taste and number of servings. We prefer twice as much celery as rice in the dish. Green peppers may be added. Tomatoes are not recommended as a suitable combination, although in the traditional dish these are used.

## Sprouting Directions

Sprouts may be made from soybeans, mung beans, grains, etc. in the following manner:

Thoroughly wash the desired material, remove broken seeds, soak overnight and place whole seeds in a perforated vessel from which all water may drain. Cover with a damp cloth and place in a dark warm room or closet. Twice each day moisten the contents by submerging in warm water. Allow to drain before returning to the darkness. These sprouts are ready for use as soon as they are ½ inch long. Sprouts will keep well in the refrigerator.

As the beans or grains sprout, the starches and proteins

are gradually converted into sugars. Therefore sprouts are classed as green vegetables and may be mixed with salad materials, or sautéed with onions and served as a vegetable or with another vegetable. Sprouts are usually an ingredient of chop suey. They may be purchased in the Chinese sections of most large cities.

### Vegetable Chop Suey

2 cups shredded Chinese cabbage
3 stalks sliced celery with tops
2 sliced onions
¼ lb. soy bean sprouts
2 cups water
1½ tbs. arrowroot or wheat flour
1 tbs. vegetable oil
1 sliced green pepper

Mix onion and celery and steam for 7 minutes. Add water and flour, and steam for 7 additional minutes. Add rest of ingredients and simmer until tender. Add oil and a little ground dulse or kelp, if desired. Serve with brown rice.

### Brown Rice Loaf

2 cups brown rice
1 bunch carrots
½ lb. string beans
2 onions
1 bunch celery

Wash rice and soak overnight in enough water to cover. Grind or grate onion, celery, string beans and carrots with skin after scrubbing them thoroughly. Mix with rice and bake for 30 minutes in oiled dish. Sprinkle paprika for color and flavor. Serve with favorite relish.

### Squash Pancakes

1 lb. squash
½ lb. parsnips
1 large onion
1 large clove of garlic
1 tbs. oil
Whole wheat bread crumbs

Grate squash, parsnips, onion and garlic. Mix with oil. Form into pancakes and roll in whole wheat bread crumbs. Bake in lightly greased pan in hot oven for 30 minutes. Bake on both sides.

## DESSERTS

### Apple Nut Whip

4 apples
1 cup seedless raisins
½ cup nut meal or ground nuts
1 tbs. honey

Core and grate apples. Sprinkle with lemon, adding honey to keep from turning color. Serve in sherbet glasses, with whole wheat or wheat germ wafers.

## Flahonse

Whole flax seed
Whole sesame seed
Honey

Mix together, unheated in equal quantities. Will keep indefinitely in any temperature. For variety, add sprinkling of carob powder or drop of genuine vanilla, or chopped dates, etc. Eat no more than 2 oz. daily.

If you prefer, the sesame and flax seed can be ground fresh and then mixed with the honey but it is best if ground with your molars.

## Blueberry Dessert

1 box blueberries or huckleberries

Wash the berries thoroughly and stew on low flame without adding any water. Takes only a few minutes to stew. Add fresh, shredded coconut or sliced bananas.

## Fruit Supreme

Equal portions of diced cantaloupe, diced honeydew melon, sliced peaches, grapes (or any other fruit or berries in season).

Serve with a dressing of sour cream and honey (to taste). Stir honey into sour cream, pour over fruit and serve with a sprinkle of wheat germ or grated nuts.

## Unbaked Fruit Loaf

¼ lb. black figs
½ lb. tart prunes

½ lb. seedless raisins
Juice of ½ lemon
¼ lb. white figs
½ lb. pitted dates
¼ lb. unsweetened, finely ground coconut

Wash prunes and remove pits. Grind fruits in food chopper. Add little honey to taste. Form into flat round or square loaf and sprinkle with coconut. Cut into layers before serving. Serve with yogurt.

### Rice Pudding

1 cup brown rice
½ cup raisins
4 tbs. of raw sugar or 6 tbs. honey
1 glass water
1½ glasses of milk
Cinnamon to flavor

Wash rice, add to boiling water and cook for 15 minutes. Add milk, raisins, sugar or honey and pour into baking dish. Bake for 45-50 minutes in moderate oven, or until brown.

### Rice and Apple Pudding

1 cup steamed brown rice
¼ cup honey
2 apples
1 quart water
1 cup seedless raisins

Steam rice in water until tender. Core and shred apples. Mix with rice, raisins and honey. Bake 25 minutes and serve. Sprinkle with wheat germ and berries or shredded coconut.

# Secrets of Health

Here are the rules for maintaining health:

*Abstain from . . .*

All processed foods
All chemically treated foods
All preserved foods
All cooked, fried, heated foods
All drugs, medicants and nostrums
All pasteurized foods
All foods containing additives or enrichments
Coffee, tea, postum, cocoa
Chocolate
Heavy protein intake
Heavy fat intake
Heavy carbohydrate intake
Chemically sprayed or dusted fruits and vegetables
Margarine
Any food containing corn syrup
Salt in any form
All foods containing baking powder or baking soda

*Eat*

A diet of practically all unfired foods
A diet consisting of green and root vegetables, grains, nuts and seeds, and fruits
Only unfluoridated or unchlorinated water wherever possible
Bread, sparingly, if you must, but only whole meal or unfragmented or untreated bread
Limited quantities of milk, butter, cheese — if you must

A good amount of daily exercise or daily physical work
Adequate sleep — 6 to 8 hours nightly

# GREYWOOD TITLE LIST